369 0127693

D1448510

This book is due for return on or before the last date shown below.

A POCKETBOOK OF

MANAGING
LOWER
BACK PAIN

WE 755 FER £21.99

For Elsevier:

Commissioning Editor: Heidi Allen, Rita Demetriou-Swanwick
Development Editor: Veronika Watkins
Project Manager: Kerrie-Anne McKinlay
Designer: Charles Gray
Illustrator: H. L. Studios
Illustrations Manager: Kirsteen Wright

A POCKETBOOK OF

MANAGING LOWER BACK PAIN

Written by

Fraser Ferguson MPhil, BSc, MCSP, SRP

Clinical Physiotherapy Specialist, Greater Glasgow Back Pain Service

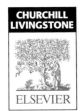

CHURCHILL LIVINGSTONE

ELSEVIER

Edinburgh London New York Oxford Philadelphia St Louis Sydney Toronto 2009

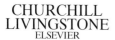

CHURCHILL
LIVINGSTONE
ELSEVIER

© 2009, Elsevier Limited. All rights reserved.

No part of this publication may be reproduced, stored in a retrieval system, or transmitted in any form or by any means, electronic, mechanical, photocopying, recording or otherwise, without the prior permission of the Publishers. Permissions may be sought directly from Elsevier's Health Sciences Rights Department, 1600 John F. Kennedy Boulevard, Suite 1800, Philadelphia, PA 19103-2899, USA: phone: (+1) 215 239 3804; fax: (+1) 215 239 3805; or, e-mail: *healthpermissions@elsevier.com*. You may also complete your request on-line via the Elsevier homepage (http://www.elsevier.com), by selecting 'Support and contact' and then 'Copyright and Permission'.

First published 2009

ISBN: 978-0-443-06846-1

British Library Cataloguing in Publication Data
A catalogue record for this book is available from the British Library

Library of Congress Cataloging in Publication Data
A catalog record for this book is available from the Library of Congress

Notice
Neither the Publisher nor the Author assume any responsibility for any loss or injury and/or damage to persons or property arising out of or related to any use of the material contained in this book. It is the responsibility of the treating practitioner, relying on independent expertise and knowledge of the patient, to determine the best treatment and method of application for the patient.

The Publisher

your source for books, journals and multimedia in the health sciences

www.elsevierhealth.com

Working together to grow libraries in developing countries

www.elsevier.com | www.bookaid.org | www.sabre.org

ELSEVIER   BOOK AID International   Sabre Foundation

The publisher's policy is to use **paper manufactured from sustainable forests**

Printed in China

Contents

Dedication **vi**

Foreword **vii**

Acknowledgements **ix**

THE PURPOSE OF THIS BOOK 1

1 REVIEW OF LOW BACK PAIN, PHYSIOTHERAPY
AND PHYSIOTHERAPISTS 5

2 IDENTIFICATION AND SIGNIFICANCE OF
RED FLAGS 21

3 IDENTIFICATION AND PHYSIOTHERAPY OF CAUDA
EQUINA SYNDROME 39

4 IDENTIFICATION AND MANAGEMENT OF
YELLOW FLAGS 51

5 THE SUBJECTIVE EXAMINATION 75

6 OBJECTIVE EXAMINATION 101

7 AN INTRODUCTION TO DIFFERENTIAL
DIAGNOSIS IN LBP PATIENTS 121

8 PAIN AND PHARMACOLOGY 143

9 PHYSIOTHERAPY TREATMENTS FOR LBP 161

10 EXAMPLES OF HOW SPECIALIST SERVICES CAN
CHANGE THE MANAGEMENT OF LBP 199

APPENDIX POSSIBLE ANSWERS TO CLINICAL
CHALLENGES AND CASE STUDIES 213

INDEX 223

Dedication

For Gillian, Rob and Jack

Foreword

It is a pleasure and a privilege to write the Foreword to this book. I sometimes wonder if there is any need for yet another book on back pain, but this is a highly original contribution that really does offer something new. It is not another textbook or a DIY manual: it is for the working therapist (physio, osteopath or chiropractor) and actually makes you think about how you manage low back pain.

This book comes from the Glasgow Back Pain Service, which is one of the most innovative and successful physiotherapy-led services for back pain in the UK. It is a thoughtful and thought-provoking little book, which reflects that background and is the product of long clinical experience and practice. The 'Clinical Challenges' are particularly useful. This is an excellent example of the modern physiotherapy approach to low back pain.

Fraser Ferguson should be congratulated on this book. I am confident you will enjoy it and that your practice will benefit from pondering on the questions he raises.

Gordon Waddell
Glasgow, July 2008

Acknowledgements

It amazes me just how good physiotherapists are now at managing low back pain rather than just trying to treat it. Either I am getting really old or the profession is starting to do something right, or both! I wrote this book based on years of clinical observations, reading, attending courses, listening to colleagues speak about back pain and patients speaking about their symptoms. In that time I have helped some patients to make themselves better, some no better and some worse!

However, I have always been fortunate enough to be part of a physiotherapy team which has a common goal. Special thanks therefore go to Mary Newton, Mick McMenemy and all my Greater Glasgow Back Pain Service colleagues, past and present, for daring to think differently about the management of low back pain in the West of Scotland.

Special thanks, too, go to Heidi Allen, Veronika Watkins and all at Elsevier for getting a rough, rambling idea of a book, full of spelling and grammatical errors, into its present form that somebody might just want to actually pick up and read!

The purpose of this book

This book has its origins in undergraduate training. As a practice educator I was always having trouble recommending relevant, practical quick reference books on the management of low back pain (LBP).

I always recommend *The Back Pain Revolution* by Gordon Waddell and continue to do so to anybody who picks up this book. *The Back Pain Revolution* is the yardstick by which all books on the lumbar spine should be compared with; it is the seminal text in the subject area with huge amounts of information. If you have never read it then do so soon (after this one of course).

This pocketbook is a very different animal. The purpose of this book is very simple: it aims to lay out all the relevant pieces that make up a low back pain (LBP) assessment from physical factors to psychosocial factors, all of which is grounded in years of clinical experience with one of the most progressive back pain services in the United Kingdom. This initial thorough assessment will give you the confidence to move on to carry out an effective treatment. It will also introduce you to clinical guidelines: why we have them, how they were developed and what ones are relevant to your clinical practice.

This book should be seen as an introductory text. *It should not be seen as a replacement for reading the other important papers and books listed throughout this book. It should not be seen as a substitute for attending credible postgraduate courses, all of which will allow you to continue to improve and fine tune your spinal assessments.* One tutor of mine suggested that every day you take something positive away from your clinical day, even if it has been the worst day with five double-bookings and nobody getting better! The positive can even be about something you have done that hasn't worked: reflecting on why it didn't work and what you might do next time is a positive learning experience. As skilled clinicians though you will have more days when more patients are getting better than worse; especially if you keep your initial LBP assessments safe and simple.

This book's prime aim is to complement what should be the ethos for the vast majority of our LBP patients...*low tech and high quality!*

Sure, a percentage of LBP will never get better; some will undergo surgery or imaging. Small numbers will attend psychology or pain management and some may require intensive physiotherapy that completely skews your monthly stats. However, most of the time following a simple but thorough assessment and initial management strategy the massive majority will improve. Let's not overcomplicate everything and make patients worse as a result.

The target audience of this book is physiotherapy students, newly qualified staff, rotational staff, and physiotherapists returning to outpatients and those with a keen interest to see if they are missing out on anything! I am sure some of you will disagree with everything I have written. Good! This can only stimulate debate and any points raised can be included in future editions. This applies to the less qualified of you who read the book and disagree or can suggest interesting additions that would enhance the text...let me know.

This book is not meant to say there is only one way to manage LBP. It's just one therapist's thoughts based on their own clinical experience and of having the pleasure of working with, discussing and sharing practice with some of the most skilled clinicians I will be likely to meet. This *expertise* is supported by some of the most up to date *evidence base* and crucially the thoughts on assessment and initial management are based on feedback from the most important part of any treatment...*the patient.*

It is not a DIY manual for LBP. Hopefully some of the content will stimulate and challenge you to discuss the points raised as well as being informative and helping you through a 'tricky' LBP assessment.

My colleagues within the Greater Glasgow Back Pain Service (GGBPS) run an introductory course to the management of LBP entitled 'Backs Aren't Scary!' They are correct – managing LBP is not scary in spite of all you may have been told. With a full carefully planned assessment, being aware of the evidence base and clinical guidelines, by recognizing red and yellow flags, by understanding basic pain mechanics you will very soon be able to carry out successful and not scary LBP assessments. Once you have this then you can carry out an equally successful and 'not scary' LBP treatment.

The term LBP used throughout this book is a generic term to signify all patients with central LBP with or without referred symptoms into the lower limb. Occasionally more specific presentations will be described and those will be clearly stated as either central LBP or leg symptoms.

Each chapter has a similar layout to give a consistent and practical feel to the pocketbook.

Clear aims and objectives are listed at the start of each chapter. It is recommended that you review these once you have finished a chapter. If you feel the text hasn't helped you meet the aims and objectives then let me know.

There are numerous CLINICAL CHALLENGES in the book. These have been designed to promote discussion and challenge your thoughts of your clinical practice.

There are also a number of CASE STUDIES based on actual patients (who have had their true identity concealed). The case studies are designed to stimulate your thought processes and put some of the information presented into some sort of clinical context.

For both of these features there are really no right or wrong answers to them. You can write answers down, just think about them or decide to ignore them.

Again, these answers are not the only answers, but will hopefully guide and prompt you in a roughly correct direction.

At the end of each chapter there are a few TAKE HOME MESSAGES that will sum up the information given and highlight the main areas of importance.

There is also a short list of recommended additional reading or places to obtain further information. This list is obviously based on my own personal preferences and is not exhaustive. However, it is an up-to-date list providing a relevant starting point to further management of LBP problems.

Review of low back pain, physiotherapy and physiotherapists

CHAPTER

1

CONTENTS

INTRODUCTION **6**

DEFINITION OF LOW BACK
PAIN (LBP) **6**

RECURRENT NATURE OF LBP **7**

TRADITIONAL PATHWAY
OF CARE **13**

CHANGING ROLE OF
PHYSIOTHERAPY IN LBP **13**

HOW DOES SELF-REFERRAL
AFFECT ME? **16**

AIMS AND OBJECTIVES

Aim: To give an overview of the incidence and the recurrent nature of low back pain (LBP) and how it has huge financial implications for health services, governments and patients

Objectives: At the end of this chapter the reader will be able to:

1. Discuss the epidemiology of LBP
2. Be aware of financial aspects of the LBP epidemic
3. Understand the recurrent nature of LBP

INTRODUCTION

From a United Kingdom (UK) National Health Service (NHS) physiotherapy perspective musculoskeletal referrals can account for up to 94% of a physiotherapist's caseload (Akpala et al 1988). More recent estimates show that this condition still makes up the vast majority of a physiotherapist's caseload today (Clemence & Seamark 2003, Parroy 2005).

The most common single musculoskeletal condition managed in the NHS by physiotherapists is LBP with figures over the last 25 years consistently showing that approximately 30% of a general outpatient physiotherapy caseload consists of LBP (CSAG 1994, Lock et al 1999, Mandiakis & Gray 2000, McKenzie 2003).

Twenty percent of patients who suffer LBP will seek NHS medical attention for it (Mandiakis & Gray 2000). The largest single professional group who treat this condition, are physio-therapists, treating approximately 1.3 million people each year in Britain (Nachemson et al 2000, Mandiakis & Gray 2000, Pengel et al 2003, Pinnington et al 2004).

DEFINITION OF LOW BACK PAIN

LBP is simply and generally defined as pain, muscle tension, or stiffness localized between the areas covered by the 12th rib and the gluteal folds, with or without leg pain (Manek & MacGregor 2005).

A more specific definition or categorization of LBP remains more elusive.

An alternative definition of LBP has been offered by one of the foremost experts on this condition who sees it as 'a 20th century medical disaster' (Waddell 2004). Quite a statement when more than three quarters of the UK population can expect to experience LBP at some point in their lifetime.

• As we are now well into the 21st century has anything changed?

CLASSIFICATION OF LBP

Classification of LBP is quite rightly seen as the 'holy grail' of LBP research.

This particular book does not contain nearly enough pages, nor my brain enough cells to begin to discuss in any great detail how to reach this aimed-for nirvana.

Ronald Donelson, Peter O'Sullivan, Robin McKenzie, Maurtis van Tulder, Shirley Sahrman are some of the most published authors in this field. Check out their very different work and conclusions as a starting point into this labyrinth of articles around classification.

However, it is still worth highlighting the importance of classification of LBP. This may be a challenge you will pick up in the future?

‼ CLINICAL CHALLENGE 1.1

1. The benefits of a successful classification system for patients with LBP are obvious! Can you suggest (a) some of these benefits; (b) some of the pitfalls of reaching consensus in this area?

2. If we cannot define LBP then how do we know how many people have LBP?

3. Is LBP for 30 minutes after cutting the hedge 'having LBP?' or is back and raging leg pain for 3 months 'having LBP?'

4. How is this information on what is seen as LBP gathered and interpreted?

5. Spend a bit of time tracking down and reviewing the first five chapters in *Rapidly Reversible Back Pain* (information further on).

THE RECURRENT NATURE OF LBP

While classification of LBP is a big topic with many different opinions and suggestions there are significant amounts of evidence to say the majority of sufferers of LBP tend to have recurrent symptoms. (Could this be another potential classification: recurrent and non-recurrent LBP?) We all have loads of patients (or as students you soon will have....bet you can't wait, eh?) who report that they have had LBP 'on and off for years'. (This phrase is used by patients almost as often as physiotherapists use the phrase 'I'll just print out some exercises'.) Strangely this evidence on the recurrent nature of LBP is not always made crystal clear in clinical guidelines produced to help manage LBP.

Previous research and clinical guidelines (see Chapter 9) have hinted that 90% of these LBP presentations are self-limiting within 6 weeks (Nachemson et al 2000, Pengel et al 2003, Pinnington et al 2004).

The remaining 10% of patients who do not improve within the 6 weeks require a disproportionate use of health services, estimated at as much as 80% of the total cost of treating LBP (Indahl et al 1995, Nachemson 1992).

The general discussion with patients is 'not to worry this problem will clear up in about 6 weeks no matter what you do'. The spin-off of this though is why bother with what treatment you do anyhow as things are clearing up so quickly?

!! **CLINICAL CHALLENGE 1.2**

What sort of things make up this 'disproportionate use of health services'?

The perception that LBP disappears from where it came is based on a lot of the evidence written down in clinical guidelines (see Chapter 9 on Clinical Guidelines for more information on this) and based on the interpretation of various epidemiological studies.

This tends to be the party line. We tell patients this a lot too. But why?

We should tell patients that 'Your LBP will clear up quickly or settle' because we want them to relax, reduce their anxiety and try to get them to focus their energies on keeping fit and active. In other words to 'normalize' things.

A big part of this normalization is also to be honest with patients. If the patient has had LBP on and off for years and you're telling them it will go away then is this adding anything new to their self management? They probably already know that.

- If the patient loses their confidence in you at this stage how will that affect their adherence to the exercise programme you will give them later?

While acute episodes do generally settle down there are huge numbers of patients for whom LBP never fully clears up.

There is sufficient evidence in the literature and anecdotally and empirically that LBP does come back with high rates of recurrence reported at around 50% (Donelson 2006, McKenzie 2003), suggesting ongoing costs to health care providers and anguish to patients too.

Because of this information it could even be suggested the challenge for those managing LBP is how to manage it effectively rather than to focus on curing it.

This crucial issue is discussed much more eloquently in the first five chapters of Ronald Donelson's book *Rapidly Reversible Low Back Pain* (2006).

- Every physiotherapist has a moral obligation to at least read these first chapters (if not the whole book) to examine just what the beast LBP actually is and how to start to tame it.

‼ CLINICAL CHALLENGE 1.3

Do you manage or help patients to manage LBP or do you try to cure patients with LBP?

Look out your notes of your last two LBP patients

What was the treatment plan and what aims for treatment were agreed?

Was this realistic? Was the plan to **cure** or **manage**?

For your next two LBP patients ask them what their expectations of physiotherapy are. How many **will say** cure me or help me self manage?

(*Continued*)

> How many **actually did say** cure me or help me self manage?
>
> How does it make you feel if you cannot cure LBP patients? I guess the answer may differ depending on (a) experience and (b) length of time qualified.

COST OF LBP

Overall, sufferers of LBP make substantial demands on the health care system, with huge costs attributable to sufferers' absence from work (CSAG 1994, Scottish Office 1998, van Tulder et al 1997).

Recent estimates within the United Kingdom (UK) suggest that 5% of LBP sufferers are absent from their work because of LBP (Department of Work and Pensions 2003).

The relevance of these changes from a physiotherapy perspective is made clearer when the estimated costs for NHS physiotherapy are reviewed. Over a decade ago estimated NHS costs were £24 to £36 million per annum (Hutchison et al 1999). More recent estimates suggest this figure is closer to £150 million (Mandiakis & Gray 2000).

In addition to NHS costs LBP has a significant impact on the work and pensions economy of the UK (CSAG 1994, Department of Work and Pensions 2003, Scottish Office 1998) with most recent estimates being thought closer to 5 billion pounds and an estimated 12% of the total numbers claiming unemployment benefits attributing their inability to work to a direct consequence of their LBP (HSE 2005).

Although these epidemiological reports failed to break down those numbers into physical and non-physical reasons for absence from work, they are still a clear indicator of the large financial implications of LBP to the UK.

Waddell (2004) notes the actual number of people claiming social security benefits because of LBP has levelled off after years of rising. Whether this change is due to improved medical intervention is less clear or as Leech (2004) proposes is due to alternative methods of dealing with disability issues, such as return to work schemes.

To assist practitioners on the most appropriate and effective healthcare for LBP, clinical guidelines based on the best available high-quality evidence and comparable with current evidence based practices, have been developed (Borkan & Cherkin 1996, Deyo 1996, Grimmer et al 2003, Koes et al 2003, Shekelle et al 1999, van Tulder et al 1997). See Chapter 9 on Clinical Guidelines for much more information on this subject.

The Royal College of General Practitioners (RCGP) Clinical Guidelines for the Management of Acute Low Back Pain (Hutchison et al 1999) are perhaps the most well known guidelines underpinning overall management and clinical practice of LBP in the United Kingdom (UK).

- The RCGP guidelines were planned to provide evidence-based recommendations for the management of LBP, in the UK, in a multidisciplinary framework that was exposed to reviews and local implementation.
- Recently the RCGP guidelines have been superseded by The Prodigy Guidelines (NHS 2005); however, both sets of guidelines strongly advocated the use of a 'diagnostic triage' in the assessment of acute LBP.
- This triage is when patients are categorized as having 'simple LBP', 'nerve root pain', or 'serious spinal pathology', with rapid access to physiotherapy for patients with acute symptoms (Hutchison et al 1999, Waddell 2004).

See Chapter 2 on red flags and Chapter 3 on cauda equina syndrome for more information on serious spinal pathology and other red flags.

OTHER COSTS OF LBP

1. Direct costs

Direct costs refer to those costs that involve money costs and commonly include costs incurred for GP visits, physiotherapy services, medication, hospital services, diagnostic testing or in many cases, cost associated with private medical insurance.

Direct costs are usually significantly less than indirect costs. Medication is often seen as the single largest direct cost averaging 13% of the total direct costs (Dagenais et al 2008).

Direct non-medical costs are those related to goods and services directly because of the illness but which are not considered to be health care related. They include, for example, travel costs to attend appointments. These expenses are easy to overlook but can really be an important source of related costs.

2. Indirect costs

Indirect costs are those reflecting the economic value of consequences for which there is no direct monetary transfer such as employment and household productivity.

(a) Work

Remember employment costs include both work absences and decreased productivity for those who continue to work despite being affected by their LBP.

Indirect costs are often more difficult to measure than direct costs, especially those related to altered productivity rather than actual absenteeism.

(b) Household productivity

In addition to lost work productivity, patients with LBP may also incur productivity losses at home if they are unable to complete routine household tasks (e.g. cleaning, cooking, playing with kids, gardening etc.).

3. Intangible costs

The third type of cost that may be considered when estimating the total cost of illness for a particular disease is termed intangible costs. These costs reflect the value of decreased enjoyment of life because of illness. However, these costs are rarely included when estimating the economic burden of LBP; a bit unfair when enjoyment should be a basic human right. Patients often feel guilty too when off work with LBP and resist encouragement to get out of the house to exercise because if they are not fit for work then they are not 'allowed' to do anything else – even if it will help them get back to normal sooner.

Looking at Mandiakis & Gray's work set out in Table 1.1 emphasizes these costs.

THE TRADITIONAL PATHWAY OF CARE FOR PATIENTS WITH LBP

Traditionally an LBP patient's journey from onset of symptoms to discharge involved many steps generally involving many unnecessary and repetitive steps (MacAuley 2004).

For example, this could mean a patient would visit their general practitioner (GP) who would then refer them on to physiotherapy.

If the patient failed to improve they would be referred back to their GP to request further investigation. This often involved a referral for orthopaedic opinion or imaging.

Invariably the orthopaedic surgeon would see no need for surgery as less than 2% of LBP require surgery in the UK and refer the patient back to physiotherapy (MacAuley 2004).

For the vast majority of patients with LBP this process was an unnecessary and unfulfilling cycle as their LBP problem invariably cleared up by the time they reached the consultant (McKenzie 2005, Mulligan 2003, Waddell 2004). See Figure 1.1.

It can be suggested that this progress was also largely passive with reduced patient responsibility (see Chapter 4 on yellow flags for more details around issues with non-mechanical issues affecting LBP).

THE CHANGING ROLE OF PHYSIOTHERAPY IN THE MANAGEMENT OF LBP

Recently there has been a change in the role of physiotherapists in their management of LBP, particularly within the UK NHS.

Table 1.1 United Kingdom breakdown of LBP costs

POPULATION	TOTAL COSTS	Direct costs		Indirect costs	
		PER CAPITA	NATIONALLY	PER CAPITA	NATIONALLY	PER CAPITA
58,970,119	£12,332,000,000	£209	£1,632,000,000	£28	£10,700,000,000	£181

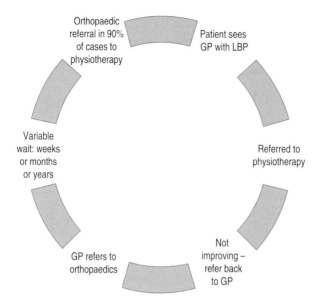

FIG 1.1 The traditional cycle of the patient with LBP.

They have been encouraged by NHS managers and politicians to work in a more autonomous and leading role taking on the parts of the role of doctors, easing pressure on services in primary care settings (CSP 2004a, Holdsworth 2004).

This is in stark comparison to the model of operation prior to the start of the increasingly autonomous physiotherapy profession whereby prior to 1975 GPs who required their patients to be seen by a physiotherapist within the NHS had to refer them to a hospital consultant who then decided on the appropriateness of the physiotherapy referral, as well as usually indicating the treatment required (Department of Health and Social Security 1977).

THANKFULLY THAT HAS CHANGED! OR HAS IT WHERE YOU WORK?

These changes to increased physiotherapy roles have been brought about through the development of clinical specialist physiotherapists, extended scope practitioners, and physiotherapy consultants all of whom could help to deliver improvements in patient care (CSP 2004).

Perhaps the biggest change in the physiotherapy role within NHS has arisen with the widespread introduction of GP- or patient-generated, self-referral to physiotherapy.

Published research in this developing field is still scarce, although there is innovative work being carried out to evaluate the benefits of this change in practice.

There is consensus in the research to date that patients who self-referred had greater compliance with attendance and lower reporting of symptom severity at follow-up, with reduced absence from work compared with those who were referred by GPs.

There was also an associated significant reduction in GP workload (Beswetherick 2003, Holdsworth & Webster 2004).

A recent follow-up to this earlier work by Holdsworth & Webster (2007) has indicated significant financial savings with patient self-referral to physiotherapy.

• The average cost of an episode of care in the NHS in the UK was
  • £66.31 for patient self-referral
  • £79.50 for a GP-suggested referral
  • £88.99 for a GP referral

All of which means that on a national scale self-referral could result in savings to NHS Scotland of approximately £2 million per annum (Holdsworth et al 2007).

HOW DOES SELF-REFERRAL AFFECT ME?

What is certain is that as a result of these changes in access and the role of physiotherapists is the responsibilities of the physiotherapy professional in regard to the management of LBP has changed for ever.

• Physiotherapists are now expected to oversee patients with LBP from onset (well not exactly from onset in an on-call type fashion, although I have spoken to a patient who phoned the physiotherapy department within 20 minutes of hurting their back!), from when a patient accesses physiotherapy through treatment and occasionally for referral to imaging, possible surgical consultation or other exit routes *often with no other GP or medical intervention.*

See Chapter 10 for examples of specialist services developed to try and re-address these issues.

- To be able to do this physiotherapists need to be aware of the current evidence for the management of LBP, current clinical guidelines for LBP, effect thorough and safe assessment of patients with LBP (see Chapter 5 on Subjective Examination and Chapter 6 on Objective Examination) and have an understanding of the many complexities and nature of the Pain part of LBP (see Chapter 8 on Pain and Pharmacology Management).

We're a small profession and we've got a big future, but are we up for the challenge?

TAKE HOME MESSAGE

Classification of LBP is the 'holy grail' of spinal care.

The problem of recurrent LBP is perhaps given less emphasis than it should. Very rarely does LBP ever go away and stay away.

LBP is a vast problem costing health care providers huge sums of money; however, an optimal treatment for it remains elusive.

How and where physiotherapists manage LBP is changing. With this increased role comes increased professional responsibility to manage it safety and effectively.

REFERENCES

Akpala C O, Curran A P, Simpson J 1988 Physiotherapy in general practice: patterns of utilisation. Public Health 102(3):263-268.

Beswetherick N 2003 Direct access to physiotherapy offers clear benefits for GPs and patients. CSP press release 17th October 2003.

Borkan J M, Cherkin D C 1996 An agenda for primary care research on low back pain. Spine 21:2880-2884.

Chartered Society of Physiotherapy 2004a Making physiotherapy count. A range of quality assured services. Chartered Society of Physiotherapy, London.

Clemence M L, Seamark D A 2003 Referring to physiotherapy or deferring? British Journal of Rehabilitation 8(4):150-154.

Clinical Standards Advisory Back Pain 1994 Report of a Clinical Standards Advisory Group on Back Pain. HMSO, London.

Dagenais S, Caro J, Haldeman S 2008 A systematic review of low back pain cost of illness studies in the United States and internationally. Spine Journal 8(91):8-20.

Department of Health and Social Security 1977 Health Service Development. Relationship between the medical and remedial professions. Health Circular 77(43).

Department of Work and Pensions 2003 Incapacity benefit days in the period 01 April 2001 to March 2002 in all areas and total for Scotland. www.dwp.gov.uk (accessed 5/11/2003).

Deyo R A, Phillips W R 1996 Low back pain: a primary care challenge. Spine 21:2826-2832.

Donelson R 2006 Rapidly Reversible Low Back Pain: Self Care First. Hanover, New Hampshire.

Grimmer K, Milanese S, Bialocerkowski A 2003 Clinical guidelines for low back pain: a physiotherapy perspective. Physiotherapy Canada (55):185-194.

Health and Safety Executive 2005 2003/4 Labour Force Survey Business http://www.hse.gov.uk/statistics/causdis/swi0304.pdf

Holdsworth L 2004 Leading professionals promote AHPs to Scottish Parliament oral evidence to the Scottish Parliament Health Committee 26/10/2004. www.csp.org.uk/scotland (last accessed 23/11/04).

Holdsworth L, Webster V 2004 Direct access to physiotherapy in primary care: now and into the future? Physiotherapy 90(2):64-72.

Holdsworth L K, Webster V S, McFadyen A K 2007 What are the costs to NHS Scotland of self-referral to physiotherapy? Results of a national trial. Physiotherapy 93:3-11.

Hutchinson A, Waddell G, Feder G 1999 Clinical guidelines for the management of acute low back pain. London: Royal College of General Practitioners; www.rcgp.org.uk (last accessed 29/08/05).

Indahl A, Velund R N, Reikeraas O 1995 Good prognosis for low back pain when left untampered. Spine 20(4):473-477.

Koes B W, van Tulder M W, Ostelo R et al 2003 Clinical guidelines for the management of low back pain in primary care: an international comparison. Spine 26:2504-2513.

Leech C 2004 The Renaissance Project, organised by the Department of Social and Family Affairs, Preventing Chronic Disability from Low Back Pain http://www.welfare.ie/publications/renaissance.html (last accessed 13/09/05).

Lock C, Allgar V, Jones K et al 1999 Prevalence of back, neck and shoulder problems in the inner city. Physiotherapy Research International 4(3):161-169.

MacAuley D 2004 Back pain and physiotherapy. BMJ 329(7468):694-695.

McKenzie R A, May S 2003 The Lumbar Spine: Mechanical Diagnosis & Therapy, 2nd Edn. Spinal Publications, Wellington.

Mandiakis N, Gray A 2000 The economic burden of back pain in the UK. Pain 84:95-103.

Manek N J, MacGregor A J 2005 Epidemiology of back disorders: prevalence, risk factors, and prognosis. Current Opinions in Rheumatology 17(2):134-140.

Mulligan J 2003 Physiotherapists working as extended scope practitioners. Physiotherapy 89(7):417–422.

Nachemson A L 1992 Newest knowledge of low back pain. Clinical Orthopaedics 279:8-20.

Nachemson A L, Waddell G, Norland A I 2000 Epidemiology of Neck and Low Back Pain. In: Nachemson A F, Jonsson E (Eds) Neck and Back Pain: The Scientific Evidence of Causes, Diagnosis, and Treatment. Lippincott Williams and Wilkins, Philadelphia.

NHS 2005 Prodigy guidance – back pain - lower www.prodigy.nhs.uk/guidance.asp?gt=Backpain-lower (accessed 10/08/05).

Parroy S 2005 The impact of allied health professionals on orthopaedic and musculoskeletal service change in Scotland. http://www.show.scot.nhs.uk/sehd/AHP/_documents/Joint%20Effects%20final.pdf (last accessed 09/01/2006)

Pengel L H M, Herbert R D, Maher C G et al 2003 Acute low back pain: systematic review of its prognosis. BMJ 327(7410):323-327.

Pinnington M A, Miller J, Stanley I 2004 An evaluation of prompt access to physiotherapy in the management of low back pain in primary care. Family Practice 21(4):372-380.

Scottish Office, Department of Health 1998 Designed to Care renewing the National Health Service in Scotland. http//www.scotland.gov.uk (last accessed 01/11/04).

Shekelle P G, Woolf S H, Eccles M et al 1999 Developing guidelines. BMJ 318:59-596.

van Tulder M W, Koes B W, Bouter L M 1997 Low back pain in primary care. Effectiveness of diagnostic and therapeutic interventions. Amsterdam: Faculteit der Geneeskunde VU. EMGO-Instituut. Cited Scher et al 2000.

Waddell G 2004 The Back Pain Revolution (2nd edn). Churchill Livingstone, Edinburgh.

Identification and significance of red flags

CHAPTER 2

CONTENTS

WHAT ARE RED FLAGS? **22**

WHAT ARE THE MOST
COMMON RED FLAGS? **25**

HOW PREVALENT ARE RED
FLAGS IN PATIENTS WITH LBP? **33**

INVESTIGATIONS – WHICH
AND WHEN? **34**

AIMS AND OBJECTIVES

Aim: To give an understanding of 'red flags' in relation to the early management of low back pain (LBP)

Objectives: At the end of this chapter the reader should be able to:

1. Define the term 'red flags'
2. Demonstrate an awareness of the significance of 'red flags' identified during physiotherapy assessment of patients with LBP
3. Demonstrate an awareness of the types of conditions to which red flags alert us
4. Identify the appropriate investigations and onward referral options available for patients presenting with 'red flags'

WHAT ARE RED FLAGS ?

With regard to low back pain red flags are: indicators of possible serious spinal pathology (Waddell 2004).

On discovering a red flag you do not necessarily need to run around panicking…however you should not ignore them either, hoping they will disappear or the GP will sort them out! The presence of red flags does not guarantee the patient has anything sinister or serious going on…….HOWEVER their absence also does not guarantee that everything is fine.

In effect, red flags **may link** a disorder to a serious pathology or severe mechanical problems.

Any identification of red flags at initial assessment should remain with the patient throughout their time under your care and should be reflected upon throughout treatment and referred to on reassessment. Equally, just because red flags are not present at the first assessment it does not mean they cannot appear at return visits to you.

The guidelines produced by the Clinical Standards Advisory Group (CSAG 1994) and Royal College of General Practitioners (Hutchinson et al 1999) recommend that in LBP a system of diagnostic triage is employed to help distinguish between them. A diagrammatic layout of this is contained in Figure 2.1 below.

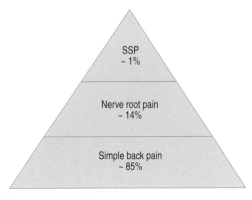

FIG 2.1 Diagnostic triage for LBP.

Simple back pain is easily the most common presentation.

The RCGP guidelines (Hutchinson et al 1999) suggest subdividing red flags into:

- Signs and symptoms requiring emergency referral:
  - Difficulty with micturition
  - Loss of sphincter tone/urinary/faecal incontinence
  - Saddle anaesthesia
  - Gait disturbance

(This area will be discussed in much more detail later in Chapter 3 on cauda equina. It is a personal opinion that although cauda equina is a red flag it is best discussed and reported on as a separate problem.)

- Signs and symptoms not requiring immediate emergency referral, which are discussed in detail in this chapter.

 CLINICAL CHALLENGE 2.1

Is this diagnostic triage an accurate example of your LBP caseload? (Fig. 2.1)

Is it fair to the huge majority of patients who have LBP of unknown origin being lumped together as just simple LBP? (See Additional Reading on Rapidly Reversible Back Pain for more information on this.)

THE SIGNIFICANCE OF INDIVIDUAL RED FLAGS FOR POSSIBLE SERIOUS SPINAL PATHOLOGY

The discovery of a red flag should be considered not on its own, but within the context of the overall clinical presentation.

It is crucial that the whole clinical picture is considered at all times. For example a patient aged 60 with long-term steroid use does not warrant immediate emergency attention, however when both are present there is a significant increased likelihood of a compression fracture being present.

Do more red flags equal more danger?

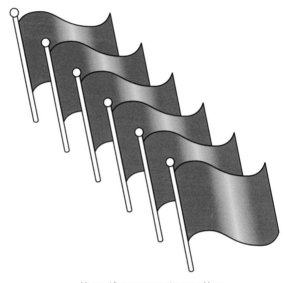

More red flags can suggest more problems

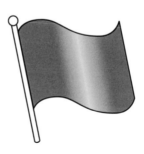

Fewer red flags can suggest fewer problems...

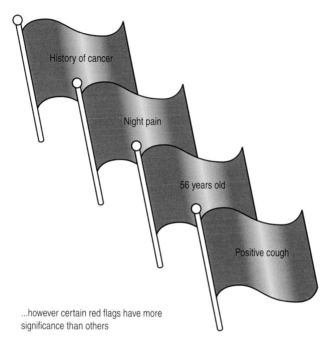

...however certain red flags have more
significance than others

Individually present factors of not responding to conservative treatment, unexplained weight loss, history of cancer or
age greater than 55 are not of major concern. However if all are
present then there is a sensitivity of nearly 100% for identifying cancer (Jarvik & Deyo 2002). In a physiotherapy setting the
vast majority of your red flags will eventually pan out as negative. However, it is not your job to diagnose red flags but highlight them, monitor and refer to the appropriate person.

WHAT ARE THE MOST COMMON RED FLAGS?

The following red flags are the most common ones you will
find in the literature (see Fig. 2.2). They are not, by any means,
agreed upon by one and all. Different clinical guidelines will list
a slightly different take on these including some but not all of
the following list. You should always be guided by your national

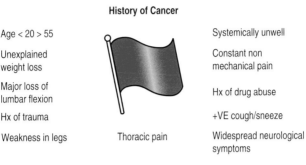

History of Cancer

Age < 20 > 55

Unexplained
weight loss

Major loss of
lumbar flexion

Hx of trauma

Weakness in legs

Thoracic pain

Systemically unwell

Constant non
mechanical pain

Hx of drug abuse

+VE cough/sneeze

Widespread neurological
symptoms

FIG 2.2 Common red flags.

and local guidelines. The following information will give you
information on why you may be asking about red flags.

AGE OF ONSET <20 OR >55

'In the young beware, in the old take care.'

In those patients younger than 20, a presentation of back pain
is more commonly associated with serious disease or a structural problem – such as spondylolisthesis.

Similarly, in those over 55 there is a much higher incidence
of serious disease (usually spinal metastasis or osteoporosis)
(Waddell 2004).

PAIN WHILE COUGHING AND/OR SNEEZING

Can you have a sore back and not have pain when you
sneeze?

Are symptoms produced or made worse when the patient
coughs and/or sneezes?

Waddell (2004) found that patients with large disc prolapse
requiring surgery had worsened symptoms when they coughed
and sneezed.

Although probably the most common and less significant
red flag, it is still best to consider it as part of the whole clinical picture. It is unlikely that postitive cough sneeze is going to
suggest a spinal tumour.

A RECENT HISTORY OF TRAUMA (E.G. A RECENT FALL OR A ROAD TRAFFIC ACCIDENT)

A normal spine is unlikely to fracture unless there is significant trauma. However, we should be aware of post-menopausal women/history of osteoporosis or those patients with a history of steroid use. Both of these conditions can weaken previously healthy bone. Also look in the next chapter about the evidence of cauda equina in patients with a history of trauma.

CONSTANT PROGRESSIVE NON-MECHANICAL PAIN

Are your symptoms constant?
Are they constant or not…they can't be both!

'Constant' means that the pain is there 24 hours every day, day and night, regardless of what the patient does or doesn't do.

Constant pain can increase or decrease in intensity but has to be there all the time.

Are symptoms and their distribution consistent with a mechanical problem? By definition a mechanical problem means that a certain movement or position can affect the pain.

Is the patient responding to treatment as you would expect? This is often known as pattern recognition, and changes as you become more experienced.

Are the symptoms mechanical, i.e. affected by movement or positioning, do symptoms vary according to activities, movements, postures, is there a pattern throughout the day? Or are they non-mechanical, i.e. there is no change to positions or movements. This may suggest a chemical or inflammatory process, which may warrant further investigations.

Are patients woken by pain and unable to get back to sleep? Does this happen every night? Nayernouri (1985 cited in Roberts) reports 'night pain relieved by walking' as an important sign to look out for.

Are the symptoms progressive, are they getting worse? Is the pain/symptoms getting more severe, is the distribution changing, are activities/function more limited? This is really closely linked to other red flags.

NIGHT PAIN

Does pain increase considerably when the patient goes to bed at night?

Constant (remember it is or isn't!) night pain is suggestive of neoplasm (Waddell 2004) but is not always present.

Night pain is not pain that is brought on when a patient is woken up while turning in bed. True night pain is pain that increases, usually severely, to such an extent that the patient has to get up from bed to seek some relief in a more upright position. An indication of true night pain is when a patient reports that the only way they can get any sleep at all is to sleep in a chair.

THORACIC PAIN

Spinal pain originating from the thoracic spine is rare; only about 2% of mechanical back problems are thoracic spine problems (McKenzie & May 2003).

Waddell (1998) has suggested that although thoracic pain is small in numbers, the seriousness of any red flags being present is large. For example 30% of patients referred to hospital with thoracic pain have serious pathology or osteoporotic collapse.

The thoracic spine is the site of primary neoplasm and secondary metastatic tumours (Boriani et al 1997, Sundaresan et al 2004), particularly those from primary sites in the prostate or breast (Tatsui et al 1996).

A Scotland-wide audit carried out by the Clinical Resource and Audit Group (CRAG) indicated that malignant cord compression is a common complication of cancer. However, this compression is frequently diagnosed late, by which time damage to the spinal cord has resulted in paraplegia.

Of particular interest to an LBP assessment is that the levels of compression as identified by MRI had very poor correspondence with the areas of pain reported by patients. Patients who presented with referred lower limb pain and neurological changes in fact had thoracic tumours. As a result of the conclusion of this widespread report the site of pain should not be used to select the level of radiological assessment, and ideally whole-spine imaging should be undertaken in all patients, whichever modality is used (CRAG 2001).

A PAST MEDICAL HISTORY OF CANCER

'Most cancer involving the spine is metastatic from the breast, lung or prostate.' (Atlas & Deyo 2001)

A previous history of cancer should always be a concern. Low back pain may present as a recurrence of a previously treated cancer, which although given the all clear has recurred, or may be the manifestation of an undiscovered problem.

Close questioning of past medical history is vital. Often, especially in the elderly, patients may not be too sure of their past medical history. Should bony metastatic secondaries be the diagnosis until ruled out?

GPs should be informed of these patients at the earliest stage for all of the above reasons if in any doubt. This is more pertinent if you are actually treating the patient and symptoms are not settling as expected….see above with regard to mechanical pain, constant, responding as you expect?

Metastases are the distant spread of cancer cells from the site of origin, which results in subsequent growth of secondary tumours (Walker 2002). The primary cancers most likely to metastasize to the bone include breast, lung, prostate, kidney and thyroid.

A primary lesion in either breast or prostate are most common areas to cause bony metastases. Primary breast, lung, prostate and kidney tumours are usually associated with spinal metastases along with multiple myelomas, lymphomas and melanomas. Spinal cord compression (SCC) that is secondary to neoplastic disease affects up to 14% of patients with metastatic disease (Garner 1999).

Lung cancer could metastasize to thoracic vertebrae in months, whereas breast cancer might take years to reach the same destination (Walker 2002).

Bone is the third most common site of metastatic disease, following the lungs and lymph nodes (Morgan 2001): the liver and brain are the next two most common sites. The spine, ribs and pelvis are commonly involved in metastatic spread, whereas the distal bones are rarely involved.

Up to 80% of patients who die of cancer have some tumour tissue in their spine. This is seen most commonly in the thoracic spine (53%) and lumbar spine (32%) (Stark et al 1982). The number of patients with a primary cancer lesion in the bone is 1% and only 0.05% with a spinal primary (Sorensen et al 1990).

From a spinal point of view, Figure 2.3 gives an interesting overview of the most common sites in the spine where cord compression as a result of serious spinal pathology can occur. This is of particular interest when you consider the information discovered by CRAG above about presentation and location not always correlating.

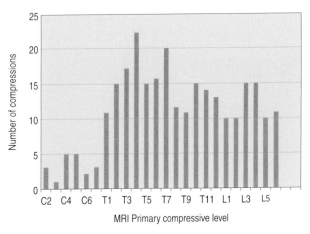

FIG 2.3 Site of spinal cord compression due to serious spinal pathology.

> **CLINICAL CHALLENGE 2.2**
>
> You have a patient with a one day history of central LBP after lifting a heavy shopping bag. She is 67 years old. Previous history of breast cancer. Pain is constant (really it is there 24 hours of the day). Patient has resorted to sleeping in an arm chair so as not to disturb her husband.
>
> What are the obvious red flags present?
>
> How worried should you be?
>
> What physiological process could be affecting symptoms at this stage?

STEROID USE

Not just in elderly or infirm, but possible in fitter athletic patients.

Patients in this group have a past medical history of long-term steroid use. Normally this is through prescribed medication for conditions such as asthma, rheumatic diseases and inflammatory bowel disease. The main relevant side affect of these medications are osteoporotic changes in the spine.

SUBSTANCE/ALCOHOL/IV DRUG ABUSE/HIV

Although not always recognized in clinical guidelines as a red flag the HIV/IVDA problem is unfortunately an increasing problem.

This can result in complications such as spinal infection which can be a major complication in patients with a history of HIV and IVDA.

Substance abuse of any kind can also result in an increased risk of trauma.

SYSTEMICALLY UNWELL

Underlying medical problems can be present at the same time as an acute episode of LBP, or may be mimicking LBP.

Malaise/fever/chills, recent infection especially skin, urinary, GI.

Other factors to be aware of are body piercing or tattoos, which can predispose to infection.

WIDESPREAD NEUROLOGICAL CHANGES

Should a neurological examination be carried out in all patients with or without referred pain (see Chapter 7 on objective examination)?

Obviously impossible if patient is not physically present. Difficult to do over the phone at a telephone triage clinic!

There is sufficient evidence to highlight patients with altered neurology as having more severe and potentially life-threatening presentation than those with minimal or no neurological changes.

Equally bilateral symptoms are often indicative of more serious spinal conditions.

Possible signs could be tripping over, legs giving way, widespread loss of sensation in legs, falls or pain in both lower limbs.

Prompt referral to a medic or physiotherapist should be considered in these patients.

WEIGHT LOSS

No history of recent weight loss does not necessarily rule out serious pathology.

In many cancers weight loss is really only evident towards the latter stages...so no weight loss reported can be a false negative...beware!

- How much weight loss is significant.........?
- Has the individual been trying to lose weight......?
- Is it because they are sore, taking medication, reduced appetite?

Atlas & Deyo (2001) define unexplained weight loss as more than 10 pounds over 6 months.

- Often patients don't always know if they have lost weight.... so ask. Do clothes still fit the same, has anybody else commented on any weight loss?

PERSISTING SEVERE LOSS OF LUMBAR FLEXION

In a study carried out by the eminent spinal authority, Professor Gordon Waddell, 50% of patients he saw in his clinic with limited lumbar flexion had either serious spinal pathology or an acute disc prolapse; 70% of patients with spinal infection had limited lumbar flexion.

Difficult to assess unless face to face. Pointers to look out for from questioning are: unable to sit down in car, home or toilet, walking all the time.

A major guiding factor in identifying these patients is if there is a structural deformity present: e.g. sciatic list/lateral shift, scoliosis, kyphosis, and spondylolisthesis.

N.B. 50% of patients reporting to a GP with back pain are not asked to undress (Waddell 2004).

 CLINICAL CHALLENGE 2.3

What other non-physical problems could result if you make too much of structural deformities? We have all had patients who have been told they have 'a twisted spine' or 'one leg longer than the other'. (See Chapter 4 for some clues.)

Remember the information at the beginning of this chapter and this doesn't mean that every patient with a severe reduction of lumbar flexion has serious pathology....it is just that patients with serious pathology tend to present with reduced flexion...a small but vital difference: *red flags are powerful tools but are only indicators of risk factors for more serious problems.*

HOW PREVALENT ARE RED FLAGS IN PATIENTS WITH LBP?

Waddell (2004) states that less than 1% of those presenting with low back pain will have a serious spinal pathology.

In Waddell's series of 900 patients consideration of 'a few key features', i.e. red flags, detected all 73 patients who had a serious spinal pathology (Waddell 2004). This was without the need for imaging, X-rays or blood tests.

McGuirk et al (2001) looked at the use of evidence-based guidelines for management of acute LBP in primary care settings and found that relying on a red flag checklist based essentially on history proved to be very safe. No red flag conditions were subsequently identified at follow-up and no serious pathologies were missed because no X-rays were taken.

Not just a financial saving but more importantly not catastrophizing what is most often a simple problem that will clear up with effective physiotherapy management.

‼ CLINICAL CHALLENGE 2.4

Your next patient with red flags:

What red flags were they?

What did you have to do?

How relevant were they to the whole clinical picture?

Are red flags exclusive to the lumbar spine?

INVESTIGATIONS – WHICH AND WHEN?

If you are worried about a patient with red flags where do they go to next? Each physiotherapy department and hospital will have their own protocols for this. The following information is a guide to what tests are most often carried out.

X-RAYS

Points to consider:
- In osteoporosis 30% of bone mass must be lost before any osteoporotic changes are seen on X-ray.
- In a cancerous lesion 50% of cancellous bone must be lost before it will show on X-ray.

That is, a patient could have had an X-ray of their lumbar spine to rule out serious spinal pathology (SSP). This has come back clear and everybody is pleased. The same patient could then have an MRI the same day, which could show SSP. A clear X-ray is a red flag red herring, a false negative.

A lumbar spine X-ray imparts 120 times the radiation of a CXR (Waddell 2004).

In the absence of red flags a 'routine' lumbar spine X-ray will pick up a serious pathology only once every 2500 X-rays (Nachemson cited in Waddell 2004).

Pain correlates poorly with the severity of degenerative change found on radiology (RCR 1993).

Repeated, regular referral for investigations such as X-ray can lead to a 'medicalization' of the problem and this is further exacerbated by diagnoses such as spondylosis or arthritis or the use of terms such as 'crumbling spine' (Deyo & Weinstein 2001).

WHEN CAN AN X-RAY BE INDICATED/NOT INDICATED?

Recommendations of clinical guidelines generally do not recommend routine plain film lumbar spine X-rays.

Clinical guidelines for LBP suggest that plain X-rays are recommended for ruling out fractures when any of the following red flags are present: recent significant trauma (any age), recent mild trauma (patient over 50), history of prolonged steroid use, osteoporosis, patient over 70.

So, basically, a lot of chat to say no to plain film X-rays as a diagnostic tool for spinal tumours! Many patients have had a clear spinal X-ray only to have a scan a short while later that shows a spine riddled with cancer.

INDICATIONS FOR MAGNETIC RESONANCE IMAGING (MRI)

- Nerve root pain not resolving with conservative treatment within 2–3 months (see Clinical Guidelines chapter)
- Progressive neurological deficit
- Cauda equina syndrome
- A known history or high-risk infection or malignancy
- MRI is the imaging means of choice (Malanga 1999)

BLOOD TESTS/URINALYSIS

There is no one specific blood test to show the presence of cancer in the spine.

Urea and electrolytes, full blood count, erythrocyte sedimentation rate and liver function test and calcium levels are the most commonly suggested but this is by no means a definitive list (Perkins et al 2003).

If in doubt.....it is always worth referring back to the patients GP and STATE your concerns. As there are so many blood tests it is always worth specifying concerns of why blood tests are being suggested i.e. possible serious spinal pathology.

TAKE HOME MESSAGE

Red flags are indicators of risk factors. They should be seen in the context of the whole clinical presentation.

Red flags should be addressed throughout the whole course of physiotherapy treatment, not just at initial assessment.

Our job as physiotherapists is not to treat red flags but refer patients to the appropriate medical professional at the appropriate time.

RECOMMENDED ADDITIONAL READING

Greenhalgh Sue, Selfe James 2006 Red Flags: A Guide to Identifying Serious Pathology of the Spine. Elsevier, Oxford.

Waddell Gordon 2004 The Back Pain Revolution, 2nd edn, chap 2. Churchill Livingstone, Edinburgh.

REFERENCES

Atlas S, Deyo R A 2001 Evaluating and managing acute low back pain in the primary care setting. Journal of General Internal Medicine 16:120-131.

Boriani S, Weinstein J N, Biagini R 1997 Primary bone tumors of the spine: terminology and surgical staging. Spine 22(9):1036-1044.

Clinical Resource and Audit Group (CRAG) 2001 A prospective audit of the diagnosis, managment and outcome of malignant cord

compression www.crag.scot.nhs.uk/committees/CEPS/reports/
F%20Report%20copy%206-2-02.PDF

Deyo R, Weinstein J N 2001 Primary care: low back pain. New
England Journal of Medicine 344(5):363-370.

Garner C 1999 Cancer-related spinal cord compression. American
Journal of Nursing 99(7):34-35.

Hutchinson A, Waddell G, Feder G 1999 Clinical guidelines for the
management of acute low back pain. Royal College of General
Practitioners, London. www.rcgp.org.uk (last accessed 29/08/05)

Jarvik J G, Deyo R A 2002 Diagnostic evaluation of low back pain with
emphasis on imaging. Annals of Internal Medicine 137(7):586-597.

McGuirk B et al 2001 Safety, efficacy and cost effectiveness of
evidence-based guidelines for the management of acute low back
pain in primary care. Spine 26(3):2615-2622.

McKenzie R A, May S 2003 The Lumbar Spine: Mechanical Diagnosis
and Therapy, 2nd edn. Spinal Publications, Wellington.

Malanga G 1999 Nonoperative treatment of low back pain. Mayo
Clinic Proceedings 74(11):1135-1148.

Morgan G 2001 Making sense of cancer. Nursing Standard 15(20):49-53.

Nachemson A Cited in Waddell 1998 The Back Pain Revolution.
Churchill Livingstone, Edinburgh.

Nayernouri T 1985 Neurilemmomas of the Cauda Equina presenting as
prolapsed lumbar intervertebral disks. Surgical Neurology 23:187-188,
cited in Roberts L 2000 Flagging the danger signs of low back pain. In:
Gifford L (ed) Topical Issues in Pain 2, CNS Press, Falmouth, p 69-83.

Perkins G L, Slater E D et al 2003 Serum tumor markers. American
Family Physician 68:1075-1082.

RCR 1993 Making the Best Use of a Department of Radiology: Guidelines
for Doctors, 2nd edn. Royal College of Radiologists, London.

Sorensen P 1990 Metastatic epidural spinal cord compression: results
of treatment and survival. Cancer 65(1):1502-1508.

Stark R 1982 Spinal metastases: a retrospective survey from a general
hospital. Brain 105(1):189-213.

Sundaresan N, Rothman A, Manhart K et al 2002 Surgery for solitary
metastases of the spine: rationale and results of treatment. Spine
27(16):1802-1806.

Tatsui H, Onomura T, Morishita S et al 1996 Survival rates of patients
with metastatic spinal cancer after scintigraphic detection of
abnormal radioactive accumulation. Spine 21(18):2143-2148.

Waddell G 2004 The Back Pain Revolution (2nd edn). Churchill
Livingstone, Edinburgh.

Walker J 2002 Caring for patients with a diagnosis of cancer and
spinal metastatic disease. Nursing Standard 16(42):41-44.

Identification and physiotherapy management of cauda equina syndrome

CHAPTER

3

CONTENTS

SETTING THE SCENE **40**

WHO GETS CES? **43**

DEVELOPMENT OF CES PATHWAY **45**

CES TRIAGE **45**

AIMS AND OBJECTIVES

Aim: To enable readers to be aware of the significance of cauda equina syndrome (CES)

Objectives: At the end of this chapter the reader should be able to:

1. Identify the signs and symptoms of patients with CES

2. Identify the signs and symptoms of CES in relation to the overall clinical presentation of patients with LBP

3. Implement the safe and effective initial management of patients with suspected CES

SETTING THE SCENE

As we have already seen LBP is the most common musculoskeletal condition managed in the NHS by physiotherapists.

- To recap: figures over the last 25 years consistently show that 20% of people who suffer LBP will seek NHS medical attention (Information Services Division (ISD) 2003, Mandiakis & Gray 2000).
- Physiotherapists are the largest single professional group who assess and manage this condition, treating approximately 1.3 million people each year in Britain (Mandiakis & Gray 2000, Nachemson et al 2000, Pinnington et al 2004).

Traditionally referrals to physiotherapy were controlled by consultants and GPs (Ferguson et al 1999). Recently in the NHS, this more traditional method has been challenged with the introduction of patient self-referral to physiotherapy (Holdsworth & Webster 2004).

As a result of the increase in physiotherapy self-referral, physiotherapists will be assessing patients sooner and in many cases without initial review by other medical professionals. This will mean physiotherapists being exposed to certain presentations of LBP which may require urgent medical attention. A prime example of one such condition is CES.

ANATOMY, STRUCTURE AND EPIDEMIOLOGY OF CES

The spinal cord tapers and ends before the first and second lumbar vertebrae, the most distal part of the cord is called the conus medullaris, and distal to this end is the collection of nerve roots know as the cauda equina (Dawodu et al 2003).

The cauda equina consists of peripheral motor and sensory nerves controlling the sensory and motor function of the lower extremities, sensation to the perineum and genitals, voluntary and involuntary functions necessary for micturition and sexual function (Nascone et al 1999).

CES occurs once the dimensions of the spinal canal are reduced beyond a critical value, at which time mechanical compression of the cauda equina nerve roots occurs (Rydevik 1993).

- Prolonged compressions of these nerves can lead to permanent disruption of these urogynaecological functions (Kennedy et al 2000, Shapiro 2000).

Figures in the literature have estimated CES as being present in 0.004% of patients with LBP (Ahn et al 2000) to 0.007% (GGBPS 2003–2006).

Although a rare complication of LBP, when CES is diagnosed it is regarded as a surgical emergency and immediate appropriate referral to accident and emergency services is necessary (Ahn et al 2000, Gleave & MacFarlane 2002, Shapiro 2000).

CAUSES OF CAUDA EQUINA SYNDROME

Central lumbar disc herniation is the most common cause of CES (Kennedy et al 2000, Shapiro 2000). Rarer causes of CES result from traumatic injury, metastatic invasion, schwannoma, pneumococcal meningitis, Paget's disease and laminar hooks (Patel 2002).

There is often a misconception among medical practitioners that CES is uniquely present in patients with acute LBP, but in approximately 70% of CES cases patients have a recent previous history of LBP (Patel 2002, Shapiro 2000).

CASE STUDY 3.1

Here is one of the most unusual cases......it is a real case. A 28-year-old man was seen at a self-referral clinic with LBP and right lower limb pain, S1 myotome and dermatome loss. Increased urinary frequency only. No saddle anaesthesia or loss of bladder/bowel control.

Physiotherapy treatment continued over a few weeks with minimal benefit. In the area this took place a specialist back pain service existed. This meant that the senior clinician

---

(Continued)

responsible for the patient was able to discuss the complex case on an ongoing basis with a local clinical physiotherapy specialist. Over the course of a week between appointments the patient suddenly developed full-blown CES. Immediate referral by local clinical physiotherapy specialist to Accident & Emergency (see later for details of pathway used). Patient had emergency discectomy. Full recovery.

The same patient 1 year later turned up at the same drop-in clinic and saw the same senior therapist. This time he was reporting a 1 month history of LBP and right lower limb pain after falling down an open manhole. No changes to bladder or bowel, continence or saddle anaesthesia were reported. As a precaution bearing in mind his previous history the patient was appointed for later that week and given clear documented instructions on what to do if he experienced any change in bladder/continence issues, using the recent previous experience as an example.

Within the space of two days between triage at drop-in clinic and full assessment the patient had developed bilateral lower limb symptoms and acute CES. He had decided not to go to A&E until a physiotherapy review. This patient was immediately referred off to A&E and next day underwent an emergency discectomy at the level below!

QUESTIONS ON CASE STUDY 3.1

(What will the patient/physiotherapist do if they ever meet at a self-referral clinic AGAIN?)

Q1.

Identify red flags from each episode.

Q2.

Was there any reason either the first or second time to refer somebody at triage with acute LBP and no clear CES symptoms straight to Accident & Emergency?

Q3.

What would you do in a similar circumstance?

I do not think anything else could have been done to prevent either surgery. There were no obvious CES symptoms at initial self-referral assessment that would merit an A & E referral.

The successful outcome I think highlights four important points:
1. Red flags should be monitored through the course of treatment…not cleared and forgotten after the first contact.
2. Patient self-referral is very effective at picking up CES. Think if the patient had waited 2 weeks for a GP appointment or had been referred as an 'urgent LBP' by his GP and sat on a waiting list for a couple of weeks.
3. An agreed pathway of care allows for a quick and streamlined referral to a surgeon, by always seeking out the advice of a more experienced colleague. (See later for an example of such a pathway for CES.)
4. Even though you feel you have given clear explict guidelines for patients to attend A&E if they develop acute CES they do not always get the message. This man even had previous experience to use as a guideline but wanted to wait until a physiotherapist had checked to make sure. Just think about how clear your message is, especially documentation in these litigious times.

WHO GETS CES?

One of the largest studies carried out on the causes of CES was reported by Ahn et al (2000). This meta-analysis reported on 322 patients with CES, of which 58% were male with an age range between 20 and 69 years. Sixty-nine percent of the patients had a sudden onset of CES. Eighty-two percent had chronic LBP for an average of 3 years before onset of CES. Trauma was associated with 62% of these cases.

SYMPTOMS AND PRESENTATION OF CES

The main symptoms suggestive of CES are:
- Saddle anaesthesia
- Increased frequency of urination
- Urinary retention
- Loss of sphincter control

WHAT ORDER DO CES SIGNS AND SYMPTOMS PRESENT IN?

Generally cauda equina syndrome develops with an increase in urinary frequency,

The next common sign is urinary retention as the bladder nerve control is compressed.

This is usually followed by frank incontinence (not stress or urge incontinence) but the first the patient is aware of this is that they are suddenly wet.
- This is like a sink overflowing if the plug is left in. There is now no bladder control to 'tell' the patient their bladder is filling up.

Saddle anaesthesia normally occurs now too. This is not an exact order but a fairly common presentation. (Gleave & MacFarlane 2002, Henriques et al 2001, Kennedy et al 2000, Patel 2002, Rydevik 1993, Shapiro 2000).

WHAT IS THE OPTIMAL TIME FOR SURGERY ON CES PATIENTS?

Assuming you discover a possible CES patient the optimal surgical intervention of patients with suspected CES is within 48 hours of onset:
- The prime reasons for earlier intervention are that sensory, motor and sphincter function are all improved by early surgical decompression, while delayed decompression can result in a poorer outcome, with reduction in full neurological function (Ahn et al 2000, Gleave & MacFarlane 2002, Henriques 2001, Kennedy et al 2000, Shapiro 2000).

These findings are of significance to physiotherapists as patients could theoretically be assessed by a physiotherapist within a day of the onset of their LBP.

DEVELOPMENT OF CES PATHWAY

One way in which there can be a more consistent approach to the early management of CES could be via the development of a city-wide pathway for managing patients with CES.

The example listed below had three components and was set up with one large urban NHS Board in Scotland.

First, a literature review was carried out. Main issues were discussed with a local neurosurgeon and as a result an evidence-based triage chart was developed and placed in every outpatient department in the city to assist physiotherapy clinicians in the initial management of suspected CES patients.

Second, a chain of communication was established to allow staff to discuss these patients with the most appropriate person.

Third, an audit cycle was developed to highlight signs and symptoms of CES and compare them with the normal population of LBP.

The whole pathway process was initiated and monitored by the clinical physiotherapy specialists working within the Greater Glasgow Back Pain Service (GGBPS), with specialist input from orthopaedic and neurosurgery consultants.

CES TRIAGE

Box 3.1 shows an overview of the triage pathway developed with three categories of urgency ranging from immediate referral to accident and emergency; careful monitoring and unlikely to be CES.

COMMUNICATION CHAIN

Central to the CES triage chart was the setting up of a chain of communication. When any outpatient physiotherapist discovered a potential CES patient they discussed the case in the first instance with the GGBPS clinical specialist physiotherapist, who in turn contacted the receiving neurosurgeon on call to discuss the case further. This chain was also an attempt to reduce unnecessary referrals direct to accident and emergency and to allow the neurosurgeon to oversee the whole referral.

AUDIT TOOL

In line with the key signs and symptoms identified from the preceding literature review an audit tool was developed by the GGBPS. These key signs were agreed by the local neurosurgeons as being appropriate to aid initial diagnosis of CES (Box 3.1).

Box 3.1 CES triage guide. Greater Glasgow back pain service CES pathway for physiotherapy management

Patients needing urgent referral to accident and emergency or neurosurgery
- Complete urinary retention
- Lack of awareness of bladder filling
- Saddle anaesthesia
- Overflow incontinence
- Saddle anaesthesia can be tested in a less invasive manner by light touch over sacral/medial gluteal area. Testing sphincter tone is not necessary
- Usually bilateral sciatica with neurological signs
- Lower limb neurological testing
- Constant non-mechanical pain
- Any recent trauma

Patients needing to be monitored
- Increased frequency
- Incontinence without saddle anaesthesia
- Whole clinical picture to be considered

Patients unlikely to have CES
- Pre-existing urological problems, e.g. history of incontinence, history of prostate problems, uterine prolapses, previous urology treatment etc…
- Incontinence due to lack of mobility
- In general these patients are aware of bladder filling but due to severe pain and fear associated with low back pain can find it difficult to reach the toilet in time
- Medication causing altered bladder/bowel function

All physiotherapists who identified a possible CES completed the audit form which reviewed presentation, duration, management and outcome of suspected CES.

OVERVIEW OF AUDIT PROCESS

The data reported on were gathered over three audit cycles. Twenty patients with suspected CES were sent to accident and emergency by following the GGBPS pathway.

The following audit information relates to the 10 patients who underwent emergency spinal surgery as a result of GGBPS pathway for CES, and offers some useful insights into important findings from your subjective and objective examination that may just help you pick up a CES patient.

RED FLAGS & CES

Patients with symptoms of CES are more likely to have a history of trauma and/or constant non-mechanical pain.

As we know from the previous chapter red flags are indicators of possible serious pathology (Waddell 2004). Table 3.1 lists the percentages of these red flags present in CES and compares them to all LBP patients from city-wide figures (GGBPS 2003–2006).

A history of trauma or constant non-mechanical pain was considerably more prevalent in patients with CES, compared with the normal population of LBP.

Table 3.1 Red flags

RED FLAG	% IN ALL LBP PATIENTS	% IN PATIENTS WITH CES
History of trauma	4%	40%
Constant non-mechanical pain	0.35%	50%
Positive cough/sneeze	21.7%	80%

NEUROLOGICAL SYMPTOMS & CES

CES patients are more likely to have multiple neurological abnormalities.

Eighty per cent of patients had more than one lower limb neurological abnormality detected, with 70% of patients having an abnormality detected in dermatome, myotome and reflex (Table 3.2).

Table 3.2 Neurological abnormalities		
NEUROLOGICAL ABNORMALITY	**% IN ALL LBP PATIENTS**	**% IN PATIENTS DIAGNOSED WITH CES**
I abnormality	40%	80%
Abnormality present in all of reflex, myotome and dermatome	20%	70%

UROLOGICAL SYMPTOMS & CES

CES patients are more likely to present with multiple urological changes.

Ninety percent of patients reported an altered from normal state of bladder or bowel function. Saddle anaesthesia was frequently present in patients with CES (80%) (Table 3.3); 70%

Table 3.3 Urological symptoms	
UROLOGICAL SYMPTOMS	**% IN PATIENTS DIAGNOSED WITH CES**
Saddle anaesthesia	90%
Retention	70%
Incontinence alone	20%
Increased frequency alone	40%
All four of the above signs	70%

TAKE HOME MESSAGE

Cauda equina syndrome (CES) is a rare complication in patients with low back pain, but when present is treated as a surgical emergency.

With the advent of patient self-referral YOU will be exposed to these patients much more often and YOU will have professional responsibility to pick these patients.

A thorough subjective examination, which considers the whole clinical picture, including a history of trauma, neurological weakness or non-mechanical pain is vital in helping recognize CES patients.

Employing a structured evidence-based pathway for patients with suspected CES can be seen as an effective and safe way in which to manage these patients.

of patients had retention or incontinence changes, and only 20% of patients reported increased urinary frequency alone. See Chapter 5 on tips for a subjective assessment tool.

RECOMMENDED READING

Ferguson F 2007 The development of a city wide pathway of care. International Journal of Therapy and Rehabilitation 14(1):24-29.

Holdsworth L, Webster V 2004 Direct access to physiotherapy in primary care: now and into the future? Physiotherapy 90(2):64–72.

Nachemson A L, Waddell G, Norlund A I 2000 Epidemiology of Neck and Low Back Pain. In: Nachemson A F, Jonsson E (eds) Neck and Back Pain: The Scientific Evidence of Causes, Diagnosis, and Treatment. Lippincott Williams & Wilkins, Philadelphia.

REFERENCES

Ahn M, Ahn N, Buchowski J et al 2000 Cauda equina syndrome secondary to lumbar disc herniation: a meta analysis of surgical outcomes. Spine 25(12):1515-1522.

Dawodu S, Lorenzo N, Kothari M 2003 Cauda equina and conus medullaris syndromes. http://www.emedicine.com/ neuro/ topic667.htm. (accessed 15/03/07)

Ferguson A, Griffin E, Mulcahy C 1999 Patient self-referral to physiotherapy in general practice: a model for the new NHS? Physiotherapy 85(1):13-20.

Gleave J R W, MacFarlane R 2002 Cauda equina syndrome: what is the relationship between timing of surgery and outcome? British Journal of Neurosurgery 16:325-328.

Greater Glasgow Back Pain Service Patient Database. Unpublished observations (2003-2006).

Henriques T, Olerud C, Pretreb-Mallmin M et al 2001 Cauda equina syndrome as a postoperative complication in five patients operated for lumbar disc herniation. Spine 3(6):293-297.

Holdsworth L, Webster V 2004 Direct access to physiotherapy in primary care: now and into the future? Physiotherapy 90(2):64-72.

Information Services Division, ISD 2003 http://www.isdscotland.org/isd/files/WFF01_ORG_040812_SH.xls (last visited 29/11/04) AHP Workforce statistics 1999-2004.

Kennedy J, Mullet H, O'Rourke K 2000 Cauda equina syndrome. Current Opinion in Orthopaedics 11:192-195.

Mandiakis N, Gray A 2000 The economic burden of back pain in the UK. Pain 84(9):95-103.

Nascone J W, Lauerman M D, Wiesel M D 1999 Cauda equina syndrome: is it a surgical emergency? Orthopaedic Journal 12(4): 73-76, University of Pennsylvania.

Patel N, Noel C, Weiner B 2002 Aortic dissection presenting as an acute cauda equina syndrome. Journal of Bone and Joint Surgery A8:1430-1432.

Pinnington M A, Miller J, Stanley I 2004 An evaluation of prompt access to physiotherapy in the management of low back pain in primary care. Family Practice 21(4):372-380.

Rydevik B 1993 Neurophysiology of cauda equina compression. Acta Orthopedic Scandinavia 64:52-55.

Shapiro S 2000 Medical realities of cauda equina syndrome secondary to lumbar disc herniation. Spine 25:348-352.

Waddell G 2004 The Back Pain Revolution (2nd Edn). Churchill Livingstone, Edinburgh.

Identification and management of yellow flags

CHAPTER

4

CONTENTS

WHAT ARE YELLOW FLAGS? **52**

MANAGEMENT OF
YELLOW FLAGS **62**

DOING SOMETHING ABOUT
YELLOW FLAGS **65**

WORDS/PHRASES TO
DISCOURAGE YELLOW FLAG
ISSUES **70**

OTHER FLAGS ASSOCIATED WITH
YELLOW FLAGS **70**

AIMS AND OBJECTIVES

Aim: To enable the reader to gain an understanding of the term 'yellow flags' and how they can affect the treatment and management of LBP

Objectives: At the end of this chapter the reader should be able to:

1. Define the term 'yellow flag'
2. Demonstrate a basic knowledge of the components that make up yellow flags
3. Recognize how yellow flags can adversely affect the management and outcomes of LBP
4. Be aware of how to begin to manage these yellow flags

WHAT ARE YELLOW FLAGS?

Yellow flags are psychosocial risk indicators that highlight the risk of developing chronic pain (Accident Compensation Corporation 2003); unlike red flags which are risk indicators of serious pathology. The presence of yellow flags does not mean the symptoms of LBP are all 'in the patient's mind'.

There are seven specific yellow flags. If you know your alphabet then they can be easily remembered; they are A, B, C, D, E, F and W (ACC 2003). If only they had come up with a yellow flag starting with 'G' to signify work then they would be even easier to remember!

ATTITUDES AND BELIEFS ABOUT BACK PAIN

These are some of the ideas and beliefs that people hold which, in themselves, can be predictors of chronic pain:

Belief that pain is harmful, resulting in fear-avoidance behaviour, guarded movements or the fear of movement, e.g. 'I am scared if I bend forward I'll never get back up'.

Belief that pain must be completely resolved before returning to work or normal daily activities and functions, e.g. 'I couldn't possibly think about going back to work until ALL my back pain has gone'.

There is the added problem that employers and those responsible for signing the patient back to work (GP) think this way too.

Worry and concern that pain will increase with work or just general activity, e.g. 'My pain will get worse if I try and get out of the house more'.

Catastrophizing, always thinking the worst, e.g. 'This pain must be something serious, could it be cancer?'.

Belief that pain is uncontrollable, e.g. 'There is nothing I can do to get relief from my pain'.

Passive attitude to rehabilitation, e.g. 'I've had acupuncture and heat numerous times before'. Did it work? 'No, but it was so relaxing, the wee physio girl was so pleasant and listened to all my worries.'

BEHAVIOURS

How patients behave in relation to back pain is very important. If they tend to sit or lie down in response to pain, this can become a habit and lead to an incorrect association between pain and rest, i.e. hurt equals harm.

The patient always needs to rest due to back pain.

Avoiding normal activity and withdrawing from day to day function or work.

Report of an extremely high intensity of pain, e.g. '20 out of 10', on a 0 to 10 Visual Analogue Scale. 'I have a high pain threshold normally.'

Has started using a stick, crutch or wheelchair.

Sleep time and quality reduced since back pain started.

COMPENSATION ISSUES

Is there any ongoing legal action against those who may have been involved in accidents?

Is there reduced financial incentive to return to work or are welfare benefits delayed or disputed over eligibility for them?

'If there's blame there's a claim' mentality, either with this episode or previous episodes. Often this is not entirely always of the patient's doing. If they are getting 'support' from a legal representative to not improve then problems may arise, especially if the 'promised' windfall entices a poor patient with significant financial rewards. I have seen an outpatient physiotherapy card that carried an advertisement for a 'if there's blame there's a claim' lawyer!

A history of prolonged periods off work due to injury or other problem, e.g. more than 12 weeks.

A history of previous back pain, with a previous claim(s) and time off work especially when linked to other points above.

DIAGNOSIS AND TREATMENT

What we say to the patient, and how we say it, is very important and can determine how they then think and behave in response to their pain.

Medical professionals encouraging prolonged disability by not providing interventions that will improve function.

A non-consistent message from the varying medical professionals who have handled the patient thus far, e.g. 'The GP told me it was sciatica, the nurse lumbago and you are saying it's a nerve root entrapment. I'm confused'.

Medical or diagnostic language leading to catastrophizing and fear, e.g. 'It's a serious disc problem you have.'

But also think how often a patient may be told 'Your X-ray looks bad. You will need to come and see me twice a week for the next three months. Can I have your credit card details please!' By now the patient is beside themselves with worry about the obvious seriousness of their problem. The X-ray shows a pelvis out of alignment, one leg is now mysteriously shorter than the other and they require 24 or so treatments and the worry that there is no way they can afford this, but if they don't pay for it then they will be unable to work anyhow and be in even more financial peril. See how easily psychosocial factors can spiral out of control with some patients?

How many times have they visited a health professional in the past for previous problems, e.g. 'The last time I was here I had acupuncture, the time before that traction, why not this time?'.

'I have sciatica'. Ask the patient what they understand by this term. What is it? Often they don't know. You can then reassure them that it is not worth being anxious and worried about something when you don't even know what it is!

An expectation of a quick-fix. 'Can't you just fix it?'. Let's be honest. Who hasn't developed pains and Googled it to get a quick fix? I had shin splints last year. I Googled it and did I click on the maintenance exercise programme hit or the one offering an instant cure? I was sore and couldn't play sport so I wanted to get better immediately and clicked on the instant cure hit. This was rationalized when I realised the instant fix would require credit card details. If there was one fix for every condition there would be far fewer hits on Google! What lengths will patients in pain go to, to be cured?

EMOTIONS

Different people respond to different stressful situations in different ways.

Fear of increased pain with activity or work.

Depression and low mood, loss of sense of enjoyment.

Increased irritability towards family and friends.

Anxiety, stress and unable to maintain sense of control.

Feelings of uselessness.

FAMILY

How other people around the patient respond to their pain plays a big role in how they then cope and manage pain.

Is there an over-protective partner at home? Although often well-intentioned, this behaviour can actually encourage catastrophizing or fear of movement.

Is the partner at home taking over tasks? e.g. 'I'm not allowed to do anything, I even get help to put on my socks'.

Worry, anxiety and fear of family members who may not be used to seeing them in such genuine severe levels of pain.

Do any family members have a history of back pain? e.g. 'My auntie Betty has had sciatica for years and is in a wheelchair now. Will I be the same?' Imagine if this is the same person with the squinty pelvis and 24 treatment recipe discussed above?

How much support family members give on any attempts to return to work.

WORK

Many issues can arise in response to a patient's ability to carry out their normal role at work.

History of heavy manual work involving significant physical demands – such as lifting, manual handling heavy items, extended periods of sitting, driving, vibration constrained or sustained postures, with an inflexible work schedule preventing appropriate breaks.

Work history, including patterns of frequent job changes, experiencing stress at work, job dissatisfaction, poor relationships with peers or supervisors.

Belief that work is harmful, unhappy at work with an absence of interest from employer or line manager.

Job involves shift work or working 'unsociable hours'.

Minimal availability and/or poor implementation of reduced duties and graduated return to work schemes.

CASE STUDY 4.1

Lesley is a 40-year-old nurse self-referred to physiotherapy with a 1-week history of LBP. It is not improving in spite of regular analgesia. This came on at work, possibly when helping a patient onto a bed in Accident and Emergency. She finished her shift but the next morning was in excruciating pain and has been off work since. At home she has stopped gardening and is spending a lot more time indoors. She is getting her husband to do most of the household chores. She is worried that if she helps out at home or does any bending her pain will never clear up. Lesley is very concerned how she will manage when she is due to return to work in 2 weeks time, especially as the department is short staffed and the nurse manager is putting a lot of pressure on staff to not take unnecessary time off. She has seen her GP for pain medication and has been told she probably has a 'slipped disc'. With her own experience of managing patients in A&E with back pain she is very aware of just how sore and debilitating this type of problem can be.

QUESTIONS ON CASE STUDY 4.1

Q1.

At what point in your assessment do you think it is appropriate to ask about yellow flags? Can yellow flags be present in patients with acute symptoms?

Q2.

What problems might you face in asking about these flags with Lesley?

Q3.

How would you put Lesley at ease while asking about yellow flags?

Q4.

What yellow flags concerning work are important to enquire about?

CHECKLIST OF QUESTIONS FOR YELLOW FLAGS

From GGBPS Yellow Flags Training Manual, 2005, with permission.

> **‼ CLINICAL CHALLENGE 4.1**
>
> For your next half dozen LBP patients make a list of any yellow flags you identified, what did you pick up on to ID them and what you are going to do to manage them. See Table 4.1 as an example. This may make more sense when you have finished this whole chapter.

Table 4.1 Yellow flag reflection chart

YELLOW FLAG PRESENT	WHAT FACTORS, PRESENTATIONS MADE YOU COME TO THAT DECISION?	PRIMARY MANAGEMENT STRATEGIES
A		
B		
C		
D		
E		
F		
W		

Pointers: ask questions as part of your normal session:
  Be INTERESTED, not ACCUSING.
  Be HONEST about your reasons for asking.

LIST OF GOOD AND NOT-SO-GOOD QUESTIONS TO ASK

The questions listed in Table 4.2 show two ways of approaching yellow flags with patients. They are not an exhaustive one; questions you may well ask are equally correct. But this table will hopefully give you some confidence to ask more and more. Can you handle the responses though?

The answers you get will help you decide whether your patient does have yellow flags in their presentation. They will also give you greater insight into the life of the patient who is coping with pain, from their point of view. If asked in the right way (respectfully and with an air of interested curiosity), they will help build a good relationship between you and the patient.

Table 4.2 A,B,C,D,E,F,W of yellow flags

ATTITUDES AND BELIEFS	BEHAVIOURS
√ Some people think pain is always a sign of damage or harm – what do you think?	√ Sometimes taking me through a typical day can help me understand things better….
√ What do you think about returning to work when in pain?	√ Can you tell me about things you have given up or do less because of the pain?
√ What do you understand is causing your pain?	√ Are there movements that cause you worry or that you steer clear of?
× What's your attitude towards the pain?	× Why have you just given up?
× Why haven't you got better?	× You must still be doing something?
× Who can get you better?	× Are you scared to move?

COMPENSATION ISSUES	DIAGNOSTIC AND TREATMENT ISSUES
√ Is there anything going on compensation- or legally-wise with you right now?	√ What do you understand is the cause of your continuing pain?
√ Are you seeking compensation for your accident at the moment?	√ Who have you seen for your pain? What have they said?
√ How is the whole legal process affecting you right now? What stage is the process at?	√ What's the best/worse advice you have received from the people you have seen?
× Why are you still seeking compensation?	× Is there any proper damage to your back?
× Does the compensation affect how much you can do?	× Haven't you been told there is nothing wrong with your back?
× Do you think it's really worth the hassle?	× I'm sure you weren't told that!

(Continued)

EMOTIONS

√ Can you tell me how your pain has affected your spirits?

√ Tell me how the pain makes you feel in your own words

√ Can your mood take a dip? Does your pain make it difficult to feel relaxed?

× Can you cheer yourself up at all?

× It's normal to feel down when you are in pain

× Has your pain affected you mentally?

FAMILY

√ What lets others know you are in more pain than normal?

√ Will your spouse do or say anything when you are in more pain?

√ How does your family feel about you doing more? What will they do when they see that?

× Do your family believe you?

× Do your family encourage you to be inactive?

× Does your spouse overprotect you?

WORK ISSUES

√ How have your employers and work colleagues been about your pain?

√ Can you tell me how things are financially at present?

√ Can you tell me what you do in your job?

× Are you going to go back to work soon?

× Don't you think it would be better to be at work than at home?

× Has your pain got worse since you've been off? Why do you think that is?

‼ CLINICAL CHALLENGE 4.2

Choose any one of the yellow flags listed in Table 4.1.

How have you asked these questions in the past? Be honest now!

CASE STUDY 4.2

Donald is a 60-year-old self-employed builder referred to physiotherapy by Accident and Emergency with 'sciatica'. He has LBP referred down the back of his right thigh for 2 months. The pain began following a busy period at work when he was working long hours to get a job done, which he hasn't managed to finish yet. Donald has been pushing himself at work to get this financially important job finished, often doubled over in pain and taking excessive medication to get by. This often results in Donald spending the weekend in bed. His mood is low and he reported having frequent arguments with his partner. Donald believed in the adage 'no pain, no gain', and was not fearful of any movement. He was confident about returning to work, but was not sure how he would achieve this on reflection. Donald felt he would be happy to work with some pain, but felt levels were too high at present to work normally.

QUESTIONS ON CASE STUDY 4.2

Q1.

How do you feel Donald might feel when you start questioning him about yellow flags?

Q2.

What yellow flags concerning behaviour would you expect to discover?

Q3.

What questions related to emotions would be important to ask about? Would this be something you would be comfortable about?

(*Continued*)

> Q4.
>
> How could you ask these to put Donald at ease?
>
> Q5.
>
> What work-related issues are important to investigate further?

MANAGEMENT OF YELLOW FLAGS

'What I think has done me the world of good in all honesty, having had a month in hospital, seeing doctors, specialists and Physiotherapists, from February I haven't seen a soul and I feel so much better.' (Patient quote from Rose, In Gifford 2002). Medicalization of pain?

'Physiotherapists are very good at identifying yellow flags, they are however less confident about their management.' (Ferguson et al 2008, Kent & Keating 2005)

WHY DO YELLOW FLAGS EXIST?

Certain factors can initiate specific beliefs about LBP and its management. What medical professionals tell the patient:

'You have a twisted spine.'

'Your discs are crumbling.'

'Looks like you have a slipped disc.'

'It's sciatica.'

How would you react if you were told any of these if you had no medical knowledge?

Is it even necessary to use these terms at all?

Does not using show we are not highly skilled and qualified practitioners?

If we don't give a diagnosis are we losing control?

Should we learn to let go?

If your average patient with LBP sees two or three different medical personnel and is told two or three different things, this usually leads to confusion and may cause unnecessary worry, behaviour and distress, i.e. YELLOW FLAGS!

What if you step outside the medical bubble for a minute......

Your car is playing up. A mechanic in the large, shiny dealership you bought the car from has told you it's one thing; a mechanic in the local, smaller one-man garage another and when you break down the RAC tells you a third reason. How do you feel? Confused, worried just how much it will cost to get better; starting to lose confidence in mechanics in general?

CASE STUDY 4.3

Jessie was referred to physiotherapy by her GP. She has turned up at the department with her son. She described experiencing back pain in her right and mid lumbar region. The pain had a tendency to settle for a few days at a time and then become severe again. Her pain is exacerbated by movements such as sneezing, coughing and laughing, with sleep regularly disturbed. This has been an ongoing problem for years and years. Apart from this Jessie is in excellent health for an 85 year old. She has no other medication and is out and about most days. Over the last week Jessie is starting to stay in more and more in case she makes her pain worse. Jessie has had numerous visits over the years to osteopaths, chiropractors and acupuncturists. They have treated her until symptoms have settled normally in three to four weeks. Jessie could only afford one visit to the chiropractor this episode. She was given an X-ray, which showed 'degenerative changes in her spine.' The chiropractor has told Jessie that she really needs an MRI to check for additional disc problems. She has asked her GP to refer her back to physiotherapy for acupuncture. Jessie's son has told her that he had some heat and

---

(Continued)

massage last year for the 'same problem' and it worked. Jessie's GP is keen to refer her to orthopaedics for an assessment too if physiotherapy doesn't work.

QUESTIONS ON CASE STUDY 4.3

Q1.

What questions relating to Jessie's beliefs about her pain would be helpful to ask?

Q2.

What questions related to behaviour are important to ask about?

Q3.

Are there any questions relating to Jessie's expectations of physiotherapy treatment that would be helpful to ask? What about her son's expectations too?

Q4.

How could you begin to explain the likely cause of Jessie's recurrent LBP?

Q5.

What might help Jessie to accept and comply with anything you do?

THE PATIENT'S PREVIOUS EXPERIENCE OF LBP

Like Jessie in Case study 4.3. She went immediately for passive therapy and got better over 4 weeks. And now you are offering an active approach to managing her LBP!

The wonders of the internet: www.curemeofallbackpain-nowandforever.com

If it's on a website it must be true mentality. Sometimes just too much information and a little knowledge can be very harmful.

THE ABILITY OF THE PATIENTS TO COPE

Depends from patient to patient. Do they lose all grip on reality when Coronation Street hasn't recorded?

This may affect how they deal with their first episode of often very, very painful LBP. No support from family, friends or work? First episode – not knowing why - catastrophic? This lack of understanding regarding LBP can easily lead to frustration mixed in with all the different messages discussed earlier. Some people do have awful lives in general. Sometimes this episode of LBP is just the final straw.

'One patient may arrive with a straightforward and realistic expectation, while another may believe that their spine is crumbling, that they will end up in a wheelchair, and that no one can do anything to prevent it. You should always try to find out what the patient expects in terms of treatment and its likely outcome.' (Waddell 2004)

HOW CAN WE BEGIN TO DO SOMETHING ABOUT YELLOW FLAGS ONCE THEY ARE IDENTIFIED?

This can be much more difficult.

It is not always easy to have your beliefs challenged. Think about it.

I used to believe that Scotland would win the 1978 World Cup. These beliefs had been built up after years of blind loyalty to my national football team and firmed up further with the hysteria before Argentina! I had these beliefs regularly challenged without any discussion or involvement by Match of the Day commentators from outwith Scotland though. I didn't like this. It made me upset and resentful. I happily joined in singing a song about one of these commentators as a result. All because my beliefs were challenged.

My beliefs about Scotland winning the World Cup have changed. Others haven't. I still believe I will shoot less than 75 for 18 holes of golf. However these beliefs are still regularly challenged from many areas. Well-meaning friends, golf coaches, family have helped re-model my own belief system that as I get older I am heading more towards the good score round the local municipal course than winning the Open Championship at St Andrews.

But think how a patient's belief system can be assaulted if you offer no build up, no reasoning or no possible solutions as part of your attempt to challenge their beliefs?

'You shouldn't slouch.'

'You should do your exercises.'

'The previous acupuncture treatment you received for your LBP, and you thought helped, won't work this time.'

How do you react? How have you reacted when you have had close beliefs, personal to you, challenged? Why should this be different for an LBP patient?

Begin to challenge negative beliefs:

Ask questions………

- 'What are you most worried about?'
- 'Is there anything that you are particularly worried about or concerned about your back pain?'
- 'What is your understanding of what is causing your back (and leg) pain?'

‼ CLINICAL CHALLENGE 4.3

Try to fit the three questions above into your next LBP assessment. They are difficult to do, but often produce interesting answers.

When you have, what sort of answers did you get?

Were you expecting these answers?

THINGS YOU MIGHT FIND HELPFUL TO SAY TO YOUR PATIENTS

'The attempt to reduce uncertainty and establish control seems to be one of the most fundamental human drives.' (Waddell 2004)

Attempt to improve the patient's knowledge regarding their back pain, thus improving their perceived control of the situation. Rather than giving them a medicalized diagnosis. Truth and honesty work in most walks of life! Why not with patients who have LBP?

FROM GGBPS *BACKS AREN'T SCARY COURSE MANUAL*, 2003 (WITH PERMISSION)

If your patient is anxious or worried, try incorporating some of the following into your assessment:

'The most important thing is to try to return to your normal activities.'

'You're doing everything you can to help your back pain.'

'What you are going through is very normal for someone suffering from LBP.'

'You have no serious pathology.' (Of course it is essential that all appropriate red flag questions are asked prior to this.)

'Less than 1% is due to serious spinal disease such as tumour or infection requiring urgent specialist investigation and treatment. Less than 1% is a systemic connective tissue disorder or inflammatory disease requiring rheumatologic investigation and treatment.' (Waddell 2004)

'Evidence suggests that those people that are fitter and more active suffer less from LBP.'

'The people who cope best with back pain are those who stay active and get on with life despite the pain.' (The Back Book 2002)

'Staying active will help you get better faster and prevent more back trouble.' (The Back Book 2002)

67

'Nerves don't tend to be trapped, they become irritated, this irritation will settle with gradually returning to normal activities.'

'Sciatica simply means pain down the back of the leg – it is a symptom, not a disease.'

'The majority of LBP is mechanical, that means certain activities tend to aggravate it, other activities tend to ease it.'…Relate this to your patient's own pain behaviour.

> **'We do not really understand the cause of most back pain and there is often very little relation between any physical pathology and the associated pain and disability.' (Waddell 2004)**

> **'Fear may become associated not only with recurrent injury, but also with pain itself. Such fears may develop into fixed beliefs about hurt and harm, and become a barrier to treatment or rehabilitation.' (Waddell 2004)**

IF YOUR PATIENT IS FEARFUL OF RETURNING TO WORK (RTW) THEN THE FOLLOWING MAY HELP BREAK DOWN ANY COMMUNICATION BARRIERS AND SHOW YOU IN A VERY EMPATHETIC LIGHT

- What are the reasons for being off work?
- Do they need to be pain-free prior to RTW?
- What are your patient's particular fears?
- Is there an opportunity for graded RTW?
- Have they been in touch with their employer?

EFFECTS OF LABELLING LBP WITH A FANCY MEDICAL DIAGNOSTIC LABEL?

> **'A slower RTW (was found in) those patients diagnosed as having sciatica or intervertebral disc problem rather**

than a non-specific diagnosis of LBP. The message for the clinician is that great care should be taken with the way in which a diagnosis is given and with the terms used.' (Watson, In Gifford 2002).

DOES YOUR PATIENT HAVE A FEAR OF RE-DAMAGING TISSUES?

Again, what are the reasons for this?
- 'The lumbar spine is one of the strongest areas of the body.'
- 'The lumbar spine likes to be moving and active.'
- 'It is better both physically and mentally to return to work and "normality".'

PATIENTS' EXPECTATIONS

'What are you expecting will help you?'
'Are you prepared to take an active part?'

Challenging your patients' negative thoughts is a relatively new thing for physiotherapists. Avoiding doing so, however, will quite likely limit the success of your management.

> *'Back pain and disability are better understood and managed as a clinical syndrome which includes important physical, psychological and social interactions.' (Rose, In Gifford 1999)*

Positive reinforcement is also very important to increase the patients' self esteem and therefore confidence. This can be done during treatments or as a consequence of setting and then achieving certain reachable goals.

Yellow flags may be present in both acute and non-acute LBP. The earlier these beliefs and behaviours are challenged, the more successful the outcome.

> *'There is now increasing evidence that these psychosocial factors are important in early stages of musculoskeletal pain.' (Watson, In Gifford 2002)*

'Early assessment and management of these (psychosocial) factors and encouragement to remain active are essential for good outcome.' (Watson, In Gifford 2002)

'Evidence has accumulated that in patients who are experiencing long term disability and who are treated with a biomedical focus (i.e. as if they had an acute episode that is going to be amenable to a 'curative' technique) the treatment may actually contribute to the ongoing disability.' (Watson & Kendall, In Gifford 2002)

SUGGESTED WORDS/PHRASES TO USE TO DISCOURAGE DEVELOPMENT OF PSYCHOSOCIAL (YELLOW FLAG) ISSUES

'Back pain is normal'/'You're in control'
'Strain/sprain', as opposed to sciatica/arthritis/derangement
'Irritation', as opposed to inflammation/trapped/pressing on
'Discomfort', as opposed to pain
'Confidence'/'movement'/'strength'/'stretch'
   Non-threatening / reassuring words…and perhaps most importantly HURT DOES NOT EQUAL HARM.

OTHER FLAGS ASSOCIATED WITH YELLOW FLAGS

In addition to yellow flags, patients can have additional blue or black flags. These are related to perceived and actual problems respectively, with a patient's occupation. Table 4.3 has a brief comparison of these.

   The management of blue and black flags is no different to the management of yellow flags in general. It is just that there will be so many more external factors influencing the outcome. Return-to-Work schemes and Occupational Health are useful contacts.

Table 4.3 Occupational flags

Yellow flags (psychosocial risk factors)	Beliefs about pain & injury (e.g. that there is a major underlying illness/disease, that avoidance of activity will help recovery, that there is a need for passive physical treatments rather than active self-management)
	Psychological distress (e.g. depression, anger, bereavement, frustration)
	Unhelpful coping strategies (e.g. fear of pain and aggravation, catastrophizing, illness behaviour, overreaction to medical problems)
	Perceived inconsistencies and ambiguities in information about the injury and its implications
	Failure to answer patients' and families' worries about the nature of the injury and its implications
Blue flags (perceived features of work or the social environment)	High demand/low control
	Unsupportive management style
	Poor social support from colleagues
	Perceived time pressure
	Lack of job satisfaction
	Work is physically uncomfortable
Black flags (not matters of perception – affect all workers equally)	Employer's rehabilitation policy deters gradual reintegration or mobility
	Threats to financial security
	Litigation/disputation over liability or contribution
	Qualification criteria for compensation (e.g. where inactivity is a qualification criterion)
	Financial incentives
	Lack of contact with the workplace
	Duration of sickness absence
	Poor co-ordination between employers and those responsible for medical care

TAKE HOME MESSAGE

Yellow flags should be addressed and managed as early as possible in patients with LBP.

Although sometimes difficult to bring up with patients, the rewards are often immeasurable in helping to achieve a mutually successful outcome to this episode of LBP. The patient very often is so relieved that a skilled practitioner has picked up on these non-mechanical issues and that they are not imagining these yellow flag symptoms.

The most important thing that can be communicated to a patient is a consistent message. This may be outwith your control at the moment as Consultants, emergency out of hours GP services, GP, alternative therapist, the internet, patients, patient's family, friends, neighbours, pets, TV doctors, soap operas... and the list goes on...who all have a different take on what is wrong. At least there is nothing stopping you as an individual therapist starting to give a consistent message to ALL your LBP patients though?

ADDITIONAL READING/INFORMATION

The following references give you a starting point to look at additional information and evidence on psychosocial yellow flags:

Linton S J 2000 Psychological Risk Factors For Neck and Back Pain. In: Nachemson A & Jonsson E (eds) Neck and Back Pain: The Scientific Evidence of Causes, Diagnosis, and Treatment. Lippincott Williams & Wilkins, Philadelphia, p 57-58.

New Zealand Guidelines Group via their web site www.nzgg.org.nz/ guidelines/dsp_guideline_popup.cfm?&guidelineID=72

REFERENCES

Accident Compensation Corporation (ACC) 2003 New Zealand Acute Low Back Pain Guide, incorporating the guide to assessing psychological yellow flags in acute low back pain. www.nzgg.og.nz/guidelines/0072/albp_guide_col.pdf (accessed 25/05/07).

Ferguson F C, Webster V, Brownlee M 2008 A Delphi study investigating consensus among expert physiotherapists in relation to the management of low back pain. Musculoskeletal Care (in press).

GGPS Backs Aren't Scarey Course Manual 2003 (Unpublished).

GGPS Yellow Flag Training Manual 2005 (Unpublished).

Gifford L S 2002 Perspectives on the biopsychosocial model–part 2. The shopping basket approach. In Touch, The Journal of the Organisation of Chartered Physiotherapist in Private Practice. Spring, issue no. 99:11-22.

Kent P, Keating J L 2005 Classification in nonspecific low back pain: what methods do primary care clinicians currently use? Spine 30(12):1433-1440.

The Back Book (2nd Edn). The Stationery Office, Norwich.

The subjective examination

CONTENTS

INTRODUCTION **76**

WHERE DO YOU START FROM? **76**

PRESENT SYMPTOMS **77**

OUTCOME MEASURES **77**

QUESTIONING **91**

AVOIDING TRAPS DURING ASSESSMENTS **95**

REFLECTIVE LISTENING **97**

AIMS AND OBJECTIVES

Aim: To enable the reader to carry out a thorough subjective examination on patients with LBP

Objectives: By the end of the chapter the reader will be able to:

1. Have sufficient knowledge to be able to carry out an effective subjective clinical examination in patients with LBP

2. Identify key subjective questioning in relation to red flags (and cauda equina)

3. Understand how the early identification of yellow flags are an integral part of any LBP assessment

4. Be aware of different types of questioning

INTRODUCTION

This chapter is not attempting to show you the only way to carry out a subjective assessment on patients with LBP. Every physiotherapist and every physiotherapy department has their own way of tackling this very important task. It is however not unfair to assume that every patient has a basic right to be asked key questions that may help identify other non-mechanical issues or may assist patients to self manage their condition in the most appropriate way.

The Chartered Society of Physiotherapy also has copious amounts of information on this subject. See Professional Standard's Number 19 on record keeping @ http://www.csp.org.uk/uploads/documents/csp_service_standards_2005.pdf

The information in this chapter will identify some of the key questions and things to look out for.

Links to other chapters will be highlighted as a pointer for more information on that area.

Depending on your own personal preferences a lot of your objective examination will be based on one type of assessment such as McKenzie's Mechanical Diagnosis and Therapy or others. The subjective is common to all.

'Patients have all the answers...do we have the right questions?' (GGBPS colleague)

WHERE DO YOU START FROM?

The self-referral clinic.

The quality of that information will vary. Although generally of a high standard, especially those screened by physiotherapists, it is your final responsibility to make sure the information is accurate and correct. Therefore it may be worthwhile to start from the very beginning as a very good place to start really.

- 'Thank you for coming.' Ever tried this as a greeting to your patients? Try it: you will be amazed at how much more positive experience your subjective examination is with this empathetic introduction.

> ## Box 5.1 WHY?
>
> Acute LBP as a condition changes rapidly, for better or worse.
> 50% of patients are never asked to undress by their GP!
> (Waddell 2004).

PRESENT SYMPTOMS

A crucially important and obvious starting point.

What symptoms does the patient have *now*.....

...not 10 years ago

...not pain from an old football injury when they hurt their knee. (This information shouldn't necessarily be ignored.... just not here though.)

But the symptoms they have at this time that prompted them to see their GP or self refer to physiotherapy.

This would normally be marked on a body chart (see Figure 5.1).

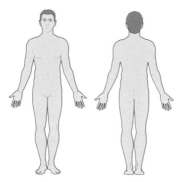

FIG 5.1 Body chart.

OUTCOME MEASURES

Any assessment should involve outcome measures. Standard 6 from the 'Standards of Physiotherapy Practice' (2005) makes an explicit requirement for members to use published, standardized outcome measures in their routine clinical practice. http://www.csp.org.uk/uploads/documents/csp_service_standards_2005.pdf

The CSP also provide a searchable outcome database. See: http://www.csp.org.uk/director/effectivepractice/outcome-measures.cfm for details.

Other examples of simpler outcome measures are:

The Visual Analogue Scale (VAS) is presented as a 10-cm line. One end is normally 'no pain' the other end 'worst imaginable pain'. You ask the patient to mark the line to indicate their present pain level. With LBP patients you may want to get them to clarify this score for any leg symptoms and central back pain. You then measure where their mark is on this line with a ruler.

0 _____ 10

Interestingly the orientation of the VAS can make a difference to the statistical distribution of any data obtained using it! Ogon et al (1996) found that data normally distributed with a horizontal VAS were abnormally distributed when the VAS was used vertically. In other words make sure your pre and post assessment is standardized!

The Numerical Rating Scale (NRS) is an 11, 21 or 101 point scale where the end points are the extremes of no pain and pain as bad as it could be, or worst pain. The NRS can be graphically or verbally delivered.

0   1   2   3   4   5   6   7   8   9   10

No matter which pain rating scale you use it is crucial that your parameters stay the same (Williamson & Hoggart 2005). For example if you ask them to rate their pain over the last week at initial assessment then this should be the parameter you use on discharge. It would also help if your departmental colleagues all agreed on the same parameters to allow more conclusive results to be drawn for an audit etc. you may carry out using these results.

What is a good aimed-for reduction in NRS/VAS? Do we need to be always looking at a 100% reduction before we can say our intervention was successful? In more acute pain this reduction is over 50% to be statistically significant (Rowbothom 2001). In chronic pain a 33% reduction is seen as statistically significant

(Rosier et al 2002). It is interesting to note that repeated VAS measurements can have a variability of up to 20%.

See Chapter 8 for more pain information.

QUEBEC TASK FORCE

In an earlier attempt to resolve the confusion over the classification of LBP the Quebec Task Force on Spinal Disorders carried out a comprehensive and critical literature review and ended up recommending the use of the classification for LBP patients (Spitzer et al 1987). (See Table 5.1.)

Table 5.1 Quebec Task Force for the classification of LBP (Spitzer 1987)

1 = Pain

2 = Pain with radiation to lower limb proximally

3 = Pain with radiation to lower limb distally

4 = Pain with radiation to lower limb and neurological signs

5 = Presumptive compression of a spinal nerve root on a simple radiogram (i.e. spinal instability or fracture)

6 = Compression of a spinal nerve root confirmed by: specific imaging techniques (computerized tomography, myelography, or magnetic resonance imaging). Other diagnostic techniques (e.g. electromyography, venography)

7 = Spinal stenosis

8 = Post surgical status, 1–6 weeks after intervention

9 = Post surgical status, >6 weeks after intervention

9.1 = Asymptomatic

9.2 = Symptomatic

10 = Chronic pain syndrome

11 = Other diagnoses

FUNCTIONAL OUTCOME MEASURE

'What one activity or movement do you find most limited by your present LBP problem?'

On discharge the patient is then asked the same question. If this activity or movement is still limited they are asked by how much.

‼ CLINICAL CHALLENGE 5.1

What do you think will be the most frequent replies to the above functional outcome measure question?

How does this outcome link to the rest of your subjective and objective assessment?

Why is it important that no matter which outcome measure you use it is applied in the same way for every patient?

Box 5.2   WHY ASK?

It is important that you at least start from the point of what relevant LBP symptoms the patient is presenting with to see you today. Patients often come with a lot of baggage that add to the holistic approach, but can often make it difficult for you to see the forest for the trees.

HOW LONG HAVE YOUR PRESENT SYMPTOMS BEEN THERE?

How long have the symptoms present today been there?
    <6 weeks equals acute
    >6 weeks equal non-acute
    Are symptoms recurrent?
    Are symptoms chronic?
Again every department will have a slightly different take on these figures, but at least this gives a starting point.

Box 5.3   WHY ASK?

This helps set the clinical presentation in front of you in some context. It allows you to honestly indicate to the patient the healing time left. It can also help in identifying issues around pain management and presentation.

See Chapter 9 for more information around this.

PRESENT SYMPTOMS CAME ON AS A RESULT OF……..?

Did the symptoms come on as a result of:
- *Trauma* (red flag)
- *Work* (yellow, blue, black flags)
- *Insidious* Figures on this are hard to find. The Greater Glasgow Back Pain Service (See Chapter 10) patient database (3000 patients over a 2-year period 2005–2007 indicates this number to be as high as 85%). This makes it very difficult for patients to proportion blame or reason with why they are just so painful and they cannot remember what they did. Discuss these facts with the patient. They are very receptive to this explanation and honesty!

Figure 5.2 gives a breakdown of how patients responded when they were asked what they thought had caused their present episode of LBP.

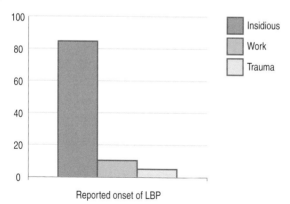

FIG 5.2 Reported means of onset of LBP (from GGBPS 2007 with permission). N = 2148.

Box 5.4   WHY ASK?

Can help to identify possible mechanisms of injury.
Highlights very important flag information.

CASE STUDY 5.1

Dave is a 41-year-old with a 2-month history of central LBP referred into his left buttock. There are no red flags or neurological deficit evident. Dave reported that his pain came on for no apparent reason. The pain is rated at 9 out of 10 on a visual analogue scale and is described as worse than when he sustained a fractured femur playing rugby 3 years ago. He cannot understand how the pain can be so severe and stopping him from carrying out normal activities of daily living when he didn't injure it. He feels he needs an X-ray or something.

QUESTIONS ON CASE STUDY 5.1

Q1.

What can you say to Dave to reassure him?

Q2.

Does he need an 'X-ray or something?'

Q3.

Describe the probable complications if Dave is not suitably reassured about his onset of LBP. How are you going to 'stop' them?

!! CLINICAL CHALLENGE 5.2

If it is so hard to find the cause of LBP and define LBP (Chapter 1), do you think it is possible to ever prevent LBP?

SYMPTOMS AT THE ONSET OF THIS EPISODE?

In this particular episode of LBP what symptoms did you have when you first noticed them?

Box 5.5   WHY ASK?

Allows you to decide whether or not there is a progressive problem that:

(a)   may need careful monitoring, e.g. central LBP at onset now referred to foot and possibly a gradually noticing weakening of ankle

(b)   may require an emergency referral, e.g. right lower limb pain, increased urinary frequency progressed to bilateral lower limb pain, saddle anaesthesia and incontinence

In many cases these questions will indicate improvements, which to a patient in pain may not be obvious and is worth explaining.

ARE SYMPTOMS INTERMITTENT OR CONSTANT?

Are symptoms there all the time? 24/7? 24 hours of every day? Or do they come and go? What positions or movements make the symptoms come or go? Sometimes patients seem to take offence at this question. It is as if they feel you don't believe them, but it is important to ask to help identify anything else going on.

Be careful that you are specific about referred symptoms i.e. central LBP increases when the patient carries out a certain movement but their leg pain is abolished. This needs to be clearly explained to a patient because to them an increasing pain is just that. They will not usually be concerned where it is increasing or if it is decreasing elsewhere.

Box 5.6   WHY ASK?

Intermittent symptoms could suggest a clear mechanical problem or directional preference.

Constant symptoms, if they are constant, can suggest maybe something more sinister, serious or a chemical pain rather than a mechanical problem.

ARE SYMPTOMS IMPROVING/UNCHANGED/ WORSENING?

Are the patient's symptoms getting better, have symptoms remained static or is there a progressive problem that may need urgent attention?

WHAT MAKES SYMPTOMS WORSE/BRINGS THEM ON OR WHAT MAKES SYMPTOMS BETTER/ABOLISHES THEM?

These questions are asked to identify any aggravating or easing factors that will affect the patient's present problem.

Also these answers can also be used to help the patient self manage their problem. Often until you ask this the patient hasn't even thought of self management. When you point out a position or movement that eases their pain they are delighted. They have a 'ground zero' exercise now; a starting point upon which to build a great self management programme. Nobody told them until you picked it up and re-packaged it in a way they could understand!!

Box 5.7   WHY ASK?

The answers to these questions are generally looked at being replicated in the objective examination.
For example a patient who complains that their LBP is made worse by sitting or bending would normally be able to reproduce their symptoms by flexing during the objective examination.
Often failure to reproduce these symptoms together with relevant red flags could indicate the need for further investigations.

When assessing the lumbar spine, the fact that some movements make things worse and some things make things better can really aid a successful outcome. This is called a DIRECTIONAL PREFERENCE. See Audrey Long's work (in the reference list) for more information on this.

‼ CLINICAL CHALLENGE 5.3

How do you know a patient is getting better?

To them it generally means a reduction in pain.

However, we know that there are many more factors that can show improvement.

Make a list of all the possible reasons a patient is 'getting better'.

To start you off: Reduced pain, increased activity, improved sleep......

How many can you get? The best list I have seen has 25 from an unnamed Queen Margaret University College undergrad. Can you beat it!

Often a patient is actually unaware that they are getting better as all they focus on is pain. Tell them about this list. It really helps both of you.

IS SLEEP DISTURBED BY THIS PRESENT PROBLEM?

This differs from night pain (see below). Sleep deprivation will make even minor pains seem so much worse to the patient.

Box 5.8   WHY ASK?

Also altered sleep postures to 'relieve' LBP can actually perpetuate the problem.

Changing to sleep in the spare room, in a bed you have not slept in before, so as not to disturb a partner can be exacerbating the problem. How many times have you been on holiday and found it takes a while to adapt to a new bed?

HAVE THERE BEEN ANY SIMILAR EPISODES OF THIS LBP OR SIMILAR PROBLEM?

IF SO WHEN?
This can indicate if the present condition is recurrent, acute, and chronic.
WHAT ABOUT THIS PREVIOUS HISTORY?
This can be very helpful in assuring the patient that things got better before. Did they require surgery, were they left with any residual problems as a result?
WHAT PREVIOUS TREATMENTS DID THEY HAVE?
Can be useful to highlight what treatments the patient had before for their LBP problem. Assuming that it will work again!

Did they remember any exercises from before? Has there been a consistent message given to the patient from other health care professionals or from previous physiotherapy assessments?

Equally it can help rationalize things for the patient. If they had a similarly severe episode 2 years ago they may have forgotten that it did actually clear up quite quickly with medication, exercise and time. Pain has made them forget this.

Reflecting on a previous episode can also be useful when the patient gets better with your successful treatment! If they are worried it will recur then you can address this anxiety by asking them to remember just how quickly they managed to clear up this episode. You have now taught them self management strategies (hopefully anyhow) on how to manage the likelihood of any recurrences…very useful.

Box 5.9   WHY ASK?

This can be a useful indicator of the possible issues around yellow flags depending on their answers or the treatment previously given.

See Chapter 4 for more information on yellow flags.

MORE SPECIFIC QUESTIONS

Box 5.10   WHY ASK?

All of these questions are related to the detection of red flags.
They are of critical importance. As the information in Chapter 3
highlighted, different red flags have different importance. It is worth
reviewing this chapter in conjunction with these questions.
It is worth remembering that in the vast majority of patients
if any red flags are present they are not related to anything
serious…….tell patients this.
You may find it worthwhile to record separately, and
highlight any red flags you have found together with possible
complications you could see arising. Makes it crystal clear when
you write so much and see so many patients.
For example:
Red flags: *Over 55 and history of trauma*
Possible complications: *Yellow flags '(work issues and reduced
L4 myotome)'*

---

*You will find that most patients come to physiotherapy and like to be
told there is nothing seriously wrong.*

COUGH/SNEEZE?

Are symptoms brought on/made worse by coughing and/or
sneezing? See Chapter 3 for more information on this subject.

BLADDER/BOWEL?

Are there any changes from the patient's NORMAL?
What is their NORMAL? Who is normal!?
   This is very difficult to skirt around. See Chapters 3 and 4 for
more information on this subject.
   • 'Have you been going to the toilet more often?'
   • 'Are you still going to the toilet regularly to pass water?'

- 'Have you had any loss of control of your bladder and/or bowel?'
- 'Have you had an accident or wet yourself?'
- 'Can you feel when you wipe between your legs?' (Either front or back areas?)

It does need to be this explicit, and is often awkward to discuss with patients.

However, this questioning is crucial to rule out any cauda equina involvement. Often the physiotherapist will rush through these questions or just move on after asking 'have there been any changes?'. Take the time to work through this list every time.

WHY THIS ORDER? See Chapter 4 for a review of this.

Look the patient straight in the eye and watch their reaction too. Often they are understandably embarrassed and may not understand.

Like any subjective questioning you need to remember your target audience.

Medical jargon is unlikely to be understood by the population in general. Working in large urban areas you will come across every kind of person, who should not be expected to understand you.

This is never more important or obvious in cauda equina questioning. To many people 'a change in frequency' is switching from Radio One FM to Radio Five Live AM.

GAIT DISTURBANCE?

Has the patient experienced any altered balance, tripping or catching of their feet? A possible indicator could suggest major neurological changes or perhaps a more central neurological problem. See Chapter 3 for more information on this subject.

PRESENT MEDICATION?

A comprehensive list of what medication prescribed, what they are actually taking. See Chapter 8 on Pain and Pharmacology. Does the patient actually know what they are taking or were prescribed?

GENERAL HEALTH?

ALMOST THREE QUARTERS of patients with LBP have co-morbid conditions (Von Korff 2005). Do we explore these enough or consider them in sufficient detail as factors for why the patient isn't getting better?

Is there any history of some (hopefully not all) of the following:

Chest problems – Is there any history of COPD? This could mean steroid use leading possibly to osteoporosis. Reduced exercise tolerance.

Angina/heart disease – Always good to know. May affect exercise regimens or referral onto exercise/back classes. Poor circulation could masquerade from a subjective point of view as referred nerve root pain.

History of stroke – Can any lower limb weakness be due to myotomal loss or stroke? Are there any residual elements from the stroke that are confusing the clinical picture, i.e. altered gait, due to CVA or serious pathology/massive disc prolapse etc?

Don't forget in all of these examples past medical history and new episodes of LBP could both be present. There is no reason a post CVA patient couldn't have left sided weakness following stroke and a large posterior-lateral disc prolapse!

Rheumatoid arthritis – History of steroids making weaker bones. Care for manual therapy techniques, osteoporotic collapse. Have they ever had a DEXA scan or test for osteoporosis?

Blood clots – Hints a poor circulation. Recent onset of calf pain following recent aeroplane flight – should you be worried?

History of cancer – See Chapter 3 for more information on this subject.

Epilepsy – Do they have it? Is it well controlled? What are their tell tale signs they are going to have an attack? Is there a person you should contact? (One patient told me that his sign that he was going to have a fit was that he went quiet and started tidying up all around him. He offered to just be left if a fit ever came on while at physiotherapy and tidy up the department.)

Diabetes – Is this type 1 (insulin dependent)? Type 2 (non-insulin dependent)?

Is this well controlled? Peripheral neuropathies can manifest or lie along side nerve root pain.

Osteoporosis – Possible indicators for referring for a DEXA scan would be (from NHS Greater Glasgow and Clyde Osteoporosis Service 2004, with permission):

- Male or female over 50 with a fracture at any site (not attributable to an RTA or fall from above head height
- Steroids >5 mg prednisolone or equivalent per day for more than 3 months
- Age 60 years + menopause aged less than 45 years
- Age >60 + acquired kyphosis
- Age >60 + significant self-reported height loss
- Age >60 years + family history of a first-degree relative with fracture (>60 at time of fracture)
- Age >60 + family history of a first-degree relative with acquired kyphosis
- Age >60 + family history of a first-degree relative with DEXA confirmed osteoporosis
- Depo Provera (Contraceptive jag) for >5 years if DEXA result will influence the use of the drug

Recent surgery – See Chapter 3 for more information on this subject.

IMAGING?

Has the patient had a recent X-ray, MRI, CT scan? This could indicate other medical problems, injury, and illness. Could be a precursor to unwittingly developing yellow flags. See Chapter 5 for non mechanical issues around this area.

HAVE THEY HAD ANY RECENT OR MAJOR SURGERY?

This can offer an insight to past medical history, fitness levels or even a potential cause for symptoms. These potential causes could range from a recent spell inactive in bed following surgery to the possibility of post operative infection. See Chapter 3 for more information on this subject.

DOES PAIN INCREASE AT NIGHT/IN BED?

Is pain becoming noticeably worse when the patient goes to bed at night? This is different to sleep being disturbed because they are sore turning or being still. Often patients with night pain report they have to sleep upright or in a chair. See Chapter 3 for more information on this subject.

HAS THE PATIENT HAD ANY RECENT FALLS, TRIPS, ACCIDENTS?

Has there been a recent history of trauma? See Chapter 2 for more information on this subject, especially non-mechanical issues around this area.

IS THERE ANY REPORTED UNEXPLAINED WEIGHT LOSS?

See Chapter 2 for more information on this subject.

QUESTIONING

The information above gives you an idea of what questions you can ask a patient with LBP.
How you ask these questions is another matter.
   It is worth your while exploring this area of questioning in more detail as there is no way in which this particular book can address the whole science of interviewing and questioning. This area is not exclusive to the management of LBP and plays a very important part in every assessment of any patient you see.
   On a very basic level there are three types of questioning:
   • Open
   • Closed
   • Leading.

OPEN QUESTIONS

An open question is asking the patient to respond to your question without any real options or limitations. For example 'Tell me what happens to your back pain when you bend forward?'.

Positives of open questions

Encourages the patient to describe their symptoms fully, without restricting their replies.

Negatives of open questions

Can lead to long-winded, non-specific responses unless well controlled.

CLOSED QUESTIONS

The patient is offered limited responses to a question. For example, 'Does bending make your back pain better or worse?' or 'Just to clarify but when you walk your leg pain is reduced?'.

Positives of closed questions

Can allow very specific answers. Useful for clarification of answers.

Negatives of closed questions

Quite restrictive.
Can be seen as limiting patients' answers.
Not overly conducive to helping the therapists with their clinical reasoning skills.

LEADING QUESTIONS

Tends to guide patients to an answer. For example: 'So bending forward will make your back pain worse?'.

Positives of leading questions

Can be useful to help clarify answers, similarly to closed questions.

Negatives of closed questions

Can lead to bias in asking questions.

Read the article by Klein (2005) in the recommended reading section for further information on how assumptions and a reliance on cognitive processes can lead to misdiagnoses.

‼ CLINICAL CHALLENGE 5.4

Open/closed/leading questions

Is this book useful to your clinical practice?

From a clinical practice point of view tell me what you think about this book.....

Tell me how you think this book will improve your clinical practice.

Obviously all the answers will be positive (another leading question!) but each question will produce varying responses. Try in your next assessment just asking open questions or closed questions. Which produced better answers to you and from a patient's perspective?

Like above the leading question assumes this book will improve your clinical practice, but doesn't give me any real feedback on how to make it better. The first question is closed and can be seen as damage limitation if I get a negative response. The second question is open and although I may get a massive answer it will be much more beneficial to let me alter change or highlight areas for future, as it will be for you to assess its usefulness or not!

CONTEXTUALIZING YOUR QUESTIONS

No matter what questions you ask it is worth remembering not to ask them as a routine list:

- 'Does bending make your LBP worse?'
- 'Does sitting make your LBP worse?'
- 'When you walk what happens to your LBP?'

A better way to ask is to put the question into some sort of context for the patient. This will lead to a better answer from which to plan your treatment and involve the patient as an equal partner in the assessment. For example:

- 'Tell me what happens to your LBP when you bend forward to pick your book off of the floor?'
- 'What happens to your LBP when you are standing in the kitchen waiting for the kettle to boil?'
- 'What would happen to your LBP if you were out walking? How long does the pain take to come on when you walk everyday to pick your son up at school?'

Similarly it is useful to use the patient's terminology. If they talk about an 'ache' rather than a 'pain' then use that terminology during the rest of the assessment – 'what happens to your ache when you….'.

…..or if they talk about a 'nervy type pain', then use that rather than changing it to your preferred terminology.

Incorporating the patient's local variances or colloquialisms on descriptions of pains into the examination is very beneficial (you may of course have to omit any expletives).

- e.g. 'Tell me what happened to that stoning pain in your back when you sit driving to work?'

It shows empathy and understanding of THEIR symptoms. Helps to establish rapport.

‼ CLINICAL CHALLENGE 5.5

Think of the times roles have been reversed. You are at the doctor, dentist, lawyer, studies advisor, clinical educator. Has every encounter gone well? Did you ever feel anxious, tense, stressed? Did you ever just agree with them just to get out???? Think about the best meetings you had. Why were they better? How did you feel?

Explore pros and cons

Try to make the patient an equal partner in the process.

Explore any discrepancies between the patient's present actual symptoms and their goals for treatment

A 40-year history of LBP and expecting to be pain-free for a wedding next week?

Assess the patient's readiness to change

Are they going to believe you and do everything you suggest, just like that with no opposition?

Assess readiness to enter treatment

Again, will they do as you suggest? It's one thing saying so in the department, just to get away from a nagging physiotherapist – but at home?

TIPS TO HELP AVOID TRAPS DURING ASSESSMENTS

The main areas of conflict during assessment are:
- Confrontation/denial trap
- Blaming trap
- Question/answer trap
- Expert trap
- Premature focus trap

Table 5.2 offers examples of how to try and avoid these traps.

THE PATIENT AND I

How often have you heard phrases like the following?
   'I think if you do your exercises………'
   'I want you to do……'

Table 5.2 Tips to help avoid traps during assessments

Confrontation/ denial trap	× A patient needs to buy into to your agreed treatment plan.	√ Arguing with someone why you really feel they should do what you are advising will simply make them more resistant to change.
Blaming trap	× Well if you did your exercises you would be better scenario. Whose 'fault' is it?	√ Did you explain them correctly? Are there other reasons for this? Discussing why and how to facilitate them is better.
Question/answer trap	× Asking questions to get the answers you want to hear and not asking questions you need to ask in case you get an answer you don't like!	√ Be careful with too many leading questions. Trust your clinical judgement and try not to lead the patient too much.
Expert trap	× A common theme of this book is that physiotherapists are experts in the management of LBP. We should not lose sight of that fact. We also don't need to remind the patient we are experts.	√ But we should also not forget that a patient is the expert in their pain. After assessment patient may think you have all the answers to their problems. √ You may not always know best for that particular patient.

| **Premature focus trap** | × | They may want nothing more than reassurance regarding serious pathology rather than a detailed list set of exercises. | √ | They may want nothing more than reassurance regarding serious pathology rather than a detailed list set of exercises Ask them, "What are you expecting from coming to physiotherapy?" Often the answers will surprise you! |

'I am going to give you……'

'I need you to do……'

It is in our nature as caring professionals who want to help their patients to slip into this terminology. We have worked hard at learning as much as we can about LBP and really need to tell the patient this….so off we go I, I, I.

While not wrong, this approach can seem very prescriptive and can exclude the patient as partner in the assessment process.

The next time you hear yourself saying 'I think….' STOP!

You will obtain far more information and adherence to treatment by asking… 'Do you think it possible that these exercises are something you could do?'.

or

'Tell me would you be able to……..'

'If I suggested……'

REFLECTIVE LISTENING

'There is no point in asking questions if you are not going to listen to the replies!'

SIMPLE REFLECTION

Patient

'The exercises do help but only at the time. I just don't have time to do them often enough. I am too busy!'

Physiotherapist

'It sounds like the exercises are helping. But it is difficult to find time to do exercises, but often it isn't the time but remembering to do them. If they are helping then maybe keeping some sort of record or set the alarm can help.'

Patient

'Right, maybe I should give it a try.'

AMPLIFIED REFLECTION

Patient

'But I can't do my exercises at home; I feel a bit embarrassed about the way I look. My kids just laugh at their mum on the floor.'

Physiotherapist

'You would be constantly feeling like your family were looking at you.'

Patient

'Well, it would be on my mind all the time. Although I really shouldn't care, as long as I was starting to see results and I am their mum!'
Forming effective reflective listening statements can help show the patient that you are tuned into what they are saying.

A bit like the information on putting their pain into a context that they understand.

Phrases you can use are:
It sounds like you…
It seems like you…
So you feel…
So you think that…
You mean that you…
You're wondering if…

Even in spite of a thorough subjective assessment identifying red flags, yellow flags, aggravating and easing factor etc. and avoiding all traps and pitfalls of entering into discussions with patients you will find out fairly soon (if you haven't already!) that you cannot make everybody better all of the time. You can only offer the facts in the best way you can.

Happily this isn't too often and the more you practice your questioning and listening techniques the less you will experience the 'you can lead the horse to water but you can't make them drink' scenario!

TAKE HOME MESSAGE

A subjective examination is a crucial first step in the assessment of LBP. Make mistakes or take short cuts here and it is likely you or the patient will pay the consequences later.

A thorough and relevant past medical history is very important. Never assume another physiotherapist or GP has covered all of this.

Outcome measures should routinely be an integral part of any examination.

Like so many things in life communication is the key. If only we spoke to each more often or listened. This is a major skill to develop. It is one that will improve every day of your clinical career if you wish it to.

RECOMMENDED ADDITIONAL READING

Farrar J T 2006 The Measurement and Analysis of Pain Symptoms. Handbook of Clinical Neurology, vol 81, chap 56 Elsevier, Oxford, p 833-842.

Klein J 2005 Five pitfalls in decisions about diagnosis and prescribing. BMJ 330:781-783.

McKenzie R M, May S 2005 The Lumbar Spine: Mechanical Diagnosis and Therapy, 2nd edn. Spinal Publications New Zealand Ltd, Wellington.

www.motivationalinterviewing.org

www.jeffallison.co.uk

www.stephenrollnick.com

REFERENCES

Chartered Society of Physiotherapy 2005 Standards of Physiotherapy Practice (SOPP).

Ogon M, Krismer M, Sollner W et al 1996 Chronic low back pain measurement with visual analogue scales in different settings. Pain 64(3):425-428.

Report of the Quebec Task Force on Spinal Disorders and an article by Spitzer et al in Spine 12(7):S1-S51.

Rosier E M, Iadarola M J, Coghill R C 2002 Reproducibility of pain measurement and pain perception. Pain 98(1&2):205-216.

Rowbotham M C 2001 What is a clinically meaningful reduction in pain? Pain 94(2):131-132.

Spitzer W O, LeBianc F E, Dupuis M et al 1987 Scientific approach to the assessment and management of activity-related spinal disorders: a monograph for clinicians report of the quebec task force on spinal disorders. Spine 12(7):S1-S51.

Spitzer W O, Skovron M L, Salmi L R et al 1995 Scientific monograph of the Quebec Task Force on whiplash-associated disorders: redefining 'whiplash' and its management. Spine 20(supplement):68S-73S.

Von Korff M, Crane P, Lane M et al 2005 Chronic spinal pain and physical-mental comorbidity in the United States: results from the national comorbidity survey replication. Pain 113(3):331-339.

Waddell G 2004 The Back Pain Revolution. Churchill Livingstone, Edinburgh.

Williamson A, Hoggart B 2005 Pain: a review of three commonly used pain rating scales. Journal of Clinical Nursing 14(7):798-804.

Objective examination

CHAPTER 6

CONTENTS

INTRODUCTION 102

OBSERVATION 104

RANGE OF MOVEMENT 105

NEUROLOGICAL EXAM 107

AIMS AND OBJECTIVES

Aim: To enable the reader to carry out a competent and relevant objective examination of the lumbar spine

Objectives: By the end of this chapter you should be able to:

1. Identify appropriate objective tests to assess LBP patients
2. Justify the choice of selected neurological tests
3. Carry out an effective neurological examination for patients with LBP
4. Identify appropriate objective markers for reassessment
5. Link objective findings to the whole clinical presentation

INTRODUCTION

Although a separate chapter, this chapter on an objective examination should always sit alongside a subjective examination. As such you should consider the information as an addition to the previous chapter and a lot of the information is interchangeable and relevant to both chapters.

A lot of the time errors, mistakes or confusion arise from newly qualified or about to be qualified physiotherapists not doing this. They are instructed to come out after the subjective examination and discuss their finding with a senior physiotherapist, before continuing with the objective examination.

This is for safety reasons and for planning and reflective purposes. But breaking it up in this way can often stop or derail the clinical reasoning process in its tracks and unconsciously limit the physiotherapist from seeing both assessments as the one important process.

This section is really a list of the most important basic objective tests you should carry out during an objective examination of the lumbar spine. Most of the time your objective assessment will follow a predetermined format depending on your undergraduate and most postgraduate training. Whether it is a McKenzie Mechanical Diagnosis and Therapy, Maitland or another format most of these objective tests will make up part or all of these assessments.

In your objective assessment you are looking at a few different things:

Red flags

See Chapter 3 for further details.

Severe LBP problems

Is there a major neurological deficit that may require referral soon to orthopaedics and or imaging?

Movement mechanics

Do the objective findings fit in with the patient's subjective reporting of their symptoms? Is there any pattern to aggravating or easing factors? You will be expecting to replicate a lot of these in the objective examination.

This can help provide you with some sort of directional preference for future treatment (Long et al 2004).

Yellow flags

Fear avoidance, exaggerated movement or responses to pain. These can become very evident in an objective examination.

Grunting and groaning during movements.

Flinching, extreme responses to pain during movement.

Fear avoidance of movement.

'I can't touch my toes at all. Can't even bend to my knees.' From a patient who is sitting comfortably in the chair or can reach their toes on long sitting.

Not actually LBP

Is it hip, thoracic, sacroiliac or something else related to the patient's past medical history or a systemic problem related to urological problems, gynaecological or rheumatologic problems? *The subjective examination should have flagged up the possibility of these being present.*

Check out the range of movement at the hip joints. Is any pain produced the 'patient's pain'?

Red flags already highlighted in subjective examination with a clear description of what aggravates and eases symptoms but on objective examination these are really mixed up, reversed, just not right no clear mechanical component.

Ask the patient! That old curve ball.

See also the following chapter for an introduction to differential diagnosis.

The patient is the expert on their pain. They will often have a fairly accurate idea of where the pain is coming from. Then when you ask actually *listen to their reply*.

- 'Where do you feel the pain is coming from?'
- 'Do you think it is your hip or your back?'
- Occasionally you are met with a 'you're the expert' reply, but more often than not you get another little nugget that will help you reach a differential diagnosis.

'You should be able to distinguish between gastrointestinal, genitourinary, hip or vascular disease, if you think about them. We miss them when we do not think, but just assume that every patient who presents with back pain must have a spinal problem.' (Waddell 2004, p 14)

OBSERVATION

Say what you see? Remember Waddell's quote. Don't be in that 50%!
Is there any *shift* or deviation from a neutral position?
Can this be corrected easily?
What happens to it when the patient lies down?

SITTING POSTURE

There is some interesting work carried out which suggests that poor posture sitting replicates itself with poor lifting postures (O'Sullivan 2007). Equally interesting is the work carried out by Wim Dankaerts et al (2006).

There was a noticeable gender difference in sitting postures. Males are much more likely to slump with their lumbar spine in flexion compared with females who tended to sit in a lordotic posture. Males sitting slumped in front of the TV or PC? Surely some major error in this study?!

Anyhow, this observation can have ramifications after your initial assessment, when you may jump into 'sit up straight' chat as part of your treatment. You may need to get females to relax into a seated position more and males to sit up straighter.

IS THERE REDUCED/INCREASED LORDOSIS?

How do you know if it is different from normal? How can you measure it? Can you measure it?

IS THERE ANY BRUISING?

This could suggest recent trauma. It could also suggest some non-mechanical component.

I can think of one patient who had seen a chiropractor before physiotherapy who presented with localized lumbar bruising for no apparent other reason than he and the chiropractor put down to being manipulated. Just didn't fit in with the whole clinical picture. Why should a big burly man with a manual job bruise so easy? Referral back to the GP for routine bloods showed an increased ESR and the patient was subsequently admitted to hospital with acute discitis.

IS THERE ANY EXAGGERATED RESPONSE TO MOVEMENT?

IS THERE ANY MUSCLE SPASM PRESENT?

What happens to it when the patient lies down?

Are there any lumps, growths, redness...*anything that doesn't fit* either with simple mechanical LBP or the subjective history?

RANGE OF MOVEMENT

> ‼ **CLINICAL CHALLENGE 6.1**
>
> Check out a model of the lumbar spine.
>
> Incidentally, does it have one of these bulging bright red disc prolapses on them?
>
> Can you imagine how a patient with acute LBP will feel when you show them this and tell them to get active??? A yellow flag catalyst if ever there was one!!

(Continued)

> Look at the facet joints? Which articular movements do they permit? How does this differ from the thoracic and cervical spines?
>
> Does the lumbar spine do more than flex and extend?

HOW TO MEASURE FLEXION AND EXTENSION

Eyeball it

0% to 100% loss. For example 0% equals no loss of movement to 100% full loss. How does this movement compare with 'normal' for the patient?

+ Easy and practical to do. Can involve the patient after carrying out the movement?

'Your range of bending forward is quite restricted. How does this compare with the amount of normal movement you have?'

+ Can be used for flexion and extension
– Very subjective

Schober's index

You mark at 5 cm below L4 to 10 cm above L4. The patient flexes and you measure the increase. A 'normal' result is an increase of more than 5 cm.

+ Recognized test for measuring lumbar mobility (Miller et al 1992)
– Palpation notoriously difficult to reproduce
– Less useful for extension

Dual inclinometer

Dual inclinometers are placed at the same starting locations on the skin. The patient is instructed to do a maximal forward flexion.

The forward flexion was measured as the difference in degrees between the pelvic and the thoraco-lumbar inclinometers with flexion (Mayer et al 1986, 1997).

+ Accurate reading of measurement
– Not every department will have one
– Placement of the goniometer needs to be accurate on repeated assessments
– Again, more difficult for measuring extension

Finger tips to the floor

You measure from the tip of the index finger to the floor. Knees kept straight. Increased movement is shown by reduced measurement.

+ Very easy to carry out. Good for patient to gauge progress on their own
– A fairly basic test. Improvements are not necessarily down to increased lumbar spine flexibility
– Once again difficult for extension

In an outpatient physiotherapy department there is no one gold standard for measuring lumbar spine range of movement. What is important is that you choose what you think is the best one for your time management; your patient group; your department and implement it as precisely as you can and try to replicate it on reassessments. There is little scientific evidence to support either methods as yet (Littlewood & May 2007).

NEUROLOGICAL EXAM

To test or not to test? That is the question!

There is a difference in opinion if neurological testing should be carried out in all LBP irrespective of whether or not they have referred pain. This difference of opinion is not exclusive to the literature base but will differ from department to department; physiotherapist to physiotherapist. A common theme running through this chapter is that there is no gold standard. Like a lot of the information, you need to reflect on what you think is the best and safest route for your patients.

Granted that carrying out too many, unnecessary, tests could perhaps cause anxiety in patients about 'what are they looking for'. But there are four good reasons that support that you always carry out a neurological examination.

1. Practice makes perfect. If you always carry out a neurological exam in every LBP patient you see then you become more proficient at it. This is important as you become more able to pick up unusual neurological responses as you have done so many 'normal' exams.

2. Provides a baseline. Either for patients whose symptoms suddenly worsen or for those who are recurrent problems. Why guess or worry over what their neurological exam was before when you can carry out a basic but very thorough exam in a few minutes?

3. Reassurance for the patient. 'I am going to carry out a few routine tests that I do on all patients with LBP.'

4. Allows important and meaningful objective markers to be integrated into your assessment. It can also allow you to show a patient when they are improving: 'Last week your muscle power was reduced....this week it is much stronger!' It is also useful to measure worsening neurological symptoms.

'WHY DO I CARRY OUT NEUROLOGICAL TESTS?'

The basic premise of any neurological exam is to differentiate between lower motor neuron involvement – that you can offer something for, or upper motor neuron involvement, which requires urgent review by a medic. See Table 6.1.

WHAT NEUROLOGICAL TESTS SHOULD I CARRY OUT?

The most common neurological tests carried out by physiotherapists with LBP are:

1. Straight leg raise
2. Reflexes

Table 6.1 Upper motor neuron involvement versus lower motor neuron involvement

	REFLEXES	MULTI-SEGMENTAL INVOLVEMENT	WEAKNESS	CLONES	UPPER LIMB INVOLVEMENT	BABINSKI
Upper motor neuron	⇑	yes	yes	yes	yes	+ve
Lower motor neuron	⇓	no	yes	×	×	−ve

3. Dermatomes
4. Myotomes

I have listed them in this particular order as an indicator of their importance in the neurological exam.

Less commonly tested are the Babinski reflex (planter reflex) and clonus test and femoral nerve stretch.

Straight leg raise (SLR)

What is it?

SLR test is a test based on stretching the nerves in the spine (Deville et al 2000).

How do I carry it out?

As there is no gold standard it is important that you choose one test and methodology and replicate it. See Figure 6.1. for one example.

It should be a passive stretch of the limb; in its most basic form it involves lifting the extended leg to a painful response

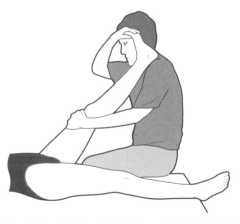

FIG 6.1 The straight leg raise. From The Physiotherapist's Pocket Book (Kenyon J & Kenyon K 2006, Churchill Livingstone, Edinburgh, Figure 1.39, p 107) with permission.

and then the knee is flexed to see if the pain goes, i.e. a positive SLR (Butler 2002).

One of the main authorities on neural tension, David Butler, devotes seven pages to the variations possible in carrying out an SLR. *Revision of these pages (pp 130–137) is strongly recommended.*

Like all neurological tests one side should be compared with the other side.

What does it show?

A very simple hypothesis is that in carrying out the SLR you are increasing the tension of the sciatic nerve that is either pushing against the protruding disc or another object (e.g. osteophyte or something more sinister) or stretching shortened scar tissue.

It could also be hypothesized that this increase in nerve tension will straighten shortened or scarred neural tissue.

Positives and negatives

+ A positive SLR is generally indicative of some underlying disc prolapse. More accurately the absence of a positive SLR suggests that it is less likely the patient has an underlying disc problem (Deville et al 2000).
+ A positive cross over SLR (SLR on the non-painful side producing pain on the other side, i.e. contralateral pain) can be seen as a strong indicator of a disc lesion (Deville at al 2000).
– Everybody does it differently and there is no gold standard of just how to do the test.
– This makes inter- and intra-assessor reliability difficult.

Reflexes

What are they and what do they show?

Deep tendon reflexes provide information on the integrity of the central and peripheral nervous system. Usually, decreased reflexes indicate a peripheral problem, i.e. caused by a nerve root lesion, and lively or exaggerated reflexes a central one.

Reflex response depends on the force of your stimulus. Use no more force than you need to provoke a definite response. Reflexes can be reinforced by having the patient perform isometric contraction of other muscles (clenched teeth, making fists).

A reduced KNEE JERK REFLEX (KJR) indicates a problem at L3/4.

A reduced ANKLE JERK REFLEX (AJR) indicates a problem at S1/S2.

How do I carry them out?

A sharp, swift tap of the patellar tendon or Achilles tendon will produce the desired response. Some studies recommend carrying these tests out in lying or with knee flexed. Often this can be difficult in elderly patients. Perhaps a solution is to carry them out with the patient sitting over the edge of the bed.

In older patients with degenerative changes affecting their knee it is often a challenge to find the patella tendon!

If you have difficulty eliciting a reflex but manage it after the umpteenth attempt it is always worth explaining this to the patient. They often get worried that it took you so long and there is something wrong!

Positives and negatives

+ Reflexes can accurately indicate nerve root compression at a level which corresponds to which reflex is reduced.
+ Brisker reflexes can indicate in some patients a more upper motor lesion. Recognized throughout the medical profession as a reliable test.
– Difficult to carry out unless practised regularly, especially at the ankle.

Dermatomes

What are they?

A dermatome is an area of *skin* that is supplied by a single pair of *dorsal roots*. See Figure 6.2.

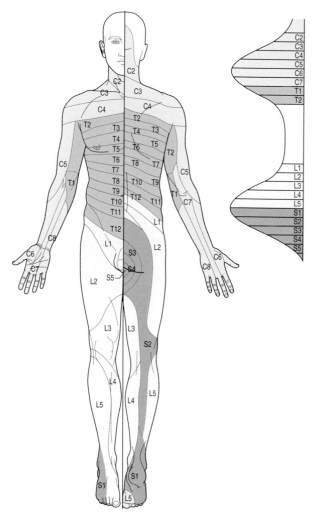

FIG 6.2 Dermatome testing. From The Physiotherapist's Pocket Book (Kenyon J & Kenyon K 2006, Churchill Livingstone, Edinburgh, Figure 1.32, p 70) with permission.

How do I carry it out?

Light touch to appropriate bilateral areas simultaneously.
Ask 'How does that feel?' Patient indicates decreased or altered sensation from *one side compared to another*.

Positives and negatives

+ Can be an accurate reflection of nerve root involvement, especially if the results fit in with additional neurological test findings and subjective reporting of site of leg symptoms.
– Patients in pain quite often experience allodynia (pain from stimuli which are not normally painful), which can confuse the picture.

Myotomes

What are they?

A myotome is used to describe the muscles served by a single spinal nerve (see Table 6.2).

What does it show?

Reduced myotomal strength can indicate a lumbar nerve root lesion.
Actual weakness in more than one muscle group could suggest other differential diagnosis (Waddell 2004).
Again, these should be looked at in context of the whole clinical picture including other neurological indicators.
Progressive myotomal weakness is often an indicator for urgent imaging/orthopaedic referral (Waddell 2004).

Positives and negatives

+ An important marker of progressive motor weakness.
– Can be the least accurate of neurological tests and patients in pain will quite often find resistance limited by pain rather than actual motor weakness?

Table 6.2 Myotome testing

NERVE ROOT	JOINT/MUSCLE ACTION	HOW TO TEST?
L2	Hip flexion	Resist hip flexion
L3	Knee extension	Resist knee extension. Remember quads are very strong weight bearing muscle; if patient able then best to check in unilateral raising from sitting (Rainville et al 2003)
L4	Dorsiflexion	Raise up onto heels and try to take a few steps
L5	Big toe extension	Resist big toe extension
S1	Heel raise	Up onto toes. Worth repeated unilaterally just to be sure
S2	Knee flexion	Resist bending the knee

Test for upper motor neuron lesions

Babinski reflex (planter reflex)

This test can be used to test for possible upper motor neuron lesions. It is carried out by a scraping stimulus along the sole of the foot.

A normal response would be flexing of the toes and evertion of the foot.

An abnormal response would be extension of the big toe and fanning of the other toes.

+ Recognized by all medical professions as a useful test for possibly identifying upper motor lesions.
− Indifferent responses are very common i.e. no response to stimulus. Skilled interpretation required (Miller et al 2005).

Clonus

If the reflexes seem hyperactive, test for ankle clonus:
1. Support the knee in a partly flexed position
2. With the patient relaxed, quickly dorsiflex the foot
3. Observe for rhythmic oscillations

Crossed adductor reflex

The patient sits with legs dangling over the edge of the bed. You strike the medical femoral condyle with the tendon hammer. A normal result will produce some contraction of the adductor muscles. An abnormal test will cause the opposite adductor tendon to contract.

Other tests

Femoral nerve stretch

A prone knee bend is carried out with the patient lying prone. This is compared to the other side.

A positive result would be anterior thigh pain. As a cautionary note PKB is starching many other tissues so accurate differential diagnosis may be difficult.

CASE STUDY 6.1

Martin is a 39-year-old musician. He has a 1-month history of LBP referred to just above the knee. This came on following a prolonged spell of sitting. Martin stood up and then bent forward to pick up his guitar case. There is no PMH of any note. There is also no past history of LBP. Sitting brings on his LBP and prolonged sitting or bending forward to pick something off the ground increases the LBP and produces the thigh pain. Martin feels his leg a bit weaker than normal walking up stairs. Objectively you have found that repeated flexion does make his symptoms worse and extension eases them considerably.

QUESTIONS ON CASE STUDY 6.1

Q1.

What neurological changes would you expect to find in Martin?

Reflexes

SLR

Dermatomes

Myotomes

Range of movement

Q2.

What other non-mechanical issues could affect the range of flexion? Why? What can you do to address these?

Just a sobering thought before the next chapter on DIFFERENTIAL DIAGNOSIS… what is the reliability of many of the physical examinations used in non-specific LBP and that you have just spent time reading in this chapter and about to read more in the next?

Funnily enough not too great. This does not mean that you should just ignore and discard the information learned/about to be learned. It's just part of the whole balancing act that is any physiotherapy assessment and treatment.

Steven May and colleagues give a really nice review of the validity and reliability of some of the most commonly used tests in the examination of LBP (see reference below). There isn't much you know!

TAKE HOME MESSAGE

An objective examination should confirm your earlier thoughts of a subjective examination.

A neurological examination in all LBP should be considered.

(Continued)

> **Practice is the key.**
>
> **Many of the objective tests have no gold standards. So choose what is the best for your particular patient group and be extra careful that you can reproduce it on reassessments and on discharge.**

RECOMMENDED ADDITIONAL READING

Butler D 2002 Mobilisation of the Nervous System. Churchill Livingstone, Edinburgh.

Deville W, van der Windt D et al 2000 The test of Lasegue. Systematic review of the accuracy in diagnosing herniated discs. Spine 25(9):1140-1147.

Littewood C, May S 2007 Measurement of range of movement in the lumbar spine – what methods are valid. A systematic review. Physiotherapy 93(3):201-211.

May S, Littlewood C, Bishop A 2006 Reliability of procedures used in the physical examination of non-specific low back pain: a systematic review. Australian Journal of Physiotherapy 52(2):91-102.

McKenzie R, May S 2003 The Lumbar Spine: Mechanical Diagnosis and Therapy, 2nd edn. Spinal Publications, Wellington.

Miller T M, Johnston S, Claiborne S 2005 Should the Babinski sign be part of the routine neurologic examination? Neurology 65(8):1165-1168.

Rainville J, Jouve C, Finno M et al 2003 Comparison of four tests of quadriceps strength in L3 or L4 radiculopathies. Spine 28(9):2466-2471.

Vlemming A, Mooney V, Stoeckart R 2007 Movement, Stability and Lumbopelvic Pain. Churchill Livingstone, Edinburgh.

REFERENCES

Butler D 2002 Mobilisation of the Nervous System. Churchill Livingstone, Edinburgh.

Dankaerts W, O'Sullivan P, Burnett A et al 2006 Differences in sitting postures are associated with nonspecific chronic low back pain disorders when patients are subclassified. Spine 31(6):698-704.

Deville W, van der Windt D et al 2000 The test of Lasegue. Systematic review of the accuracy in diagnosing herniated discs. Spine 25(9):1140-1147.

Long A, Donelson R, Fung T 2004 Does it matter which exercise? A randomized control trial of exercise for low back pain. Spine 29(23):2593-2602.

Mayer T G, Kondraske G, Beals S B et al 1997 Spinal range of motion. Accuracy and sources of error with inclinometric measurement. Spine 22:1976-1984.

Miller S A, Mayer T, Cox R et al 1992 Reliability problems associated with the modified Schober technique for true lumbar flexion measurement. Spine 17:345-348.

Miller T M, Johnston Claiborne S 2005 Should the Babinski sign be part of the routine neurologic examination? Neurology 65(8):1165-1168.

O'Sullivan P B, Dankaerts W, Burnett A F et al 2007 Effect of different upright sitting postures on spinal-pelvic curvature and trunk muscle activation in a pain-free population. Spine 31(19):E707-712.

Rainville J, Jouve C, Finno M et al 2003 Comparison of four tests of quadriceps strength in L3 or L4 radiculopathies. Spine 28(21):2466-2471.

An introduction to differential diagnosis in LBP patients

CONTENTS

POSSIBLE ERRORS IN
CLINICAL DIAGNOSIS **122**

DIFFERENTIAL DIAGNOSIS OF
LEG PAIN **124**

DIFFERENTIAL DIAGNOSIS OF
REFERRED LEG PAIN **124**

LUMBAR SPINE PAIN AND
PELVIC GIRDLE PAIN **129**

SPINAL STENOSIS **133**

SACROILIAC JOINT PAIN AND
LUMBAR SPINE PAIN **135**

FACET OR ZYGAPOPHYSEAL
JOINTS **140**

AIMS AND OBJECTIVES

Aim: To provide the reader with some of the different tests you can employ as part of your spinal examination to assist in reaching an informed differential diagnosis.

Objectives: By the end of the chapter the reader will be able to:

1. Understand the importance of not shoe-horning patients with LBP into a diagnostic box
2. Demonstrate different tests you could employ to help differentiated between spinal pain originating in the lumbar spine and sacroiliac joint
3. Have an understanding of the different common signs and symptoms of pain originating in the lumbar spine and pelvic pain
4. Demonstrate an increased awareness of the importance of differential diagnosis in the lumbar spine

A few cautionary words! Differential diagnosis is the process whereby you weigh up the probability of one structure versus another as being the most likely cause of your patient's symptoms (Figure 7.1). *It is not a flow chart or algorithm to a diagnosis. Follow that route and you will make errors.*

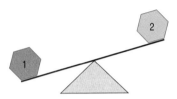

FIG 7.1 Weighing up your differential diagnosis.

POSSIBLE ERRORS IN CLINICAL DIAGNOSIS

Often as clinicians we make errors. (Surely not!!)

Everybody does! It is recognizing them and learning from them by reflecting on where we went wrong that should drive our clinical development, in the same way that reflecting on a successful outcome does.

A few of the most common pitfalls in clinical decision making are listed below. The following information is worth exploring before we move onto some differential diagnosis tests. Some of them have very grand names to explain some fairly simple principles that you might not already know that you already know them!

THE REPRESENTATIVENESS HEURISTIC

This is when you assume that a clinical presentation is similar to other things in a certain category. For example the last patient you saw with referred lower limb pain responded to extension in lying with the differential diagnosis of a prolapsed intervertebral disc. The next patient in the cubicle is telling you a similar story and their initial presentation seems to represent an identical diagnosis.

The likelihood is that perhaps this common presentation will produce an equally common differential diagnosis but not always! Often you will use this 'situational information' without enough factual information (Klein 2005).

AVAILABILITY HEURISTIC

When we use the availability heuristic, we place particular weight on examples of things that come to mind easily.

'I've just been on a course and they mentioned such and such condition and this new patient looks like they have it. Easy.'

Or 'I've just read this new fabby LBP assessment book and it says......so this patient must have it.'

This error is because these things are easily remembered or have been recently encountered. To avoid this mistake think of ALL the massive number of factors that could influence your diagnosis or clinical decision.

• Easily available information doesn't always equal relevant information.

OVERCONFIDENCE

Don't be overconfident in your assessment. This error is caused when we make a mistake in our diagnosis, perhaps not knowing our limitations. This overconfidence is particularly evident when clinicians are rushed into a quick assessment. Be aware of your limitations at any grade and spend time asking colleagues for their opinion (Koriat et al 1980).

CONFIRMATORY BIAS

Confirmatory bias is the tendency to look for, notice, and remember information that fits with our pre-existing expectations. This means that your assessment may be biased by what you found earlier in the assessment.

For example your LBP patient tells you their pain is made worse when they sit, your objective assessment may already be biased towards finding pain in flexion. The problem with this error is you may jump to a conclusion as to the cause of the symptoms. This becomes even more of a problem as treatment progresses.

Keep thinking of reasons on where the patient's symptoms may be coming from, are there possible other causes than those you thought of originally?

ILLUSORY CORRELATION

Illusory correlation happens when two actions are perceived as being related, when in fact the connection between them is coincidental or even non-existent. For example, after giving a treatment to an LBP patient you notice a splendid improvement in their symptoms. You then assume the reason for this improvement was due to the action of your treatment. However, this is not necessarily true. Is there an evidence base behind the treatment you carried out? Could your treatment have had a physiological response to the patient? Was it the treatment carried out or just the fact that you showed concern? Often you *REMEMBER* a positive outcome to a previous treatment.

- Carrying on treating patients with this illusion can in time lead to a strengthening of incorrect beliefs and suboptimal clinical practices.

DIFFERENTIAL DIAGNOSIS OF LEG PAIN

A clear pattern of the likely cause of leg pain becomes very clear during a subjective and objective assessment.

Patients with leg pain are often in high distress as is the newly qualified physiotherapist! Leg pain should be considered in tandem with the information contained in Chapter 2 on Red Flags and Chapter 8 on Pain and Pharmacology.

INTRODUCTION TO DIFFERENTIAL DIAGNOSIS OF REFERRED LEG PAIN

There are three possible *mechanical* causes of referred leg pain (Painting 1993, McKenzie & May 2003):

1. Derangement
2. Adherent nerve root
3. Nerve root entrapment

Derangement

A posterolateral displacement of disc nuclear material within an intact annulus. This is normally reducible by physiotherapy.

Entrapment

Nerve root is compromised by immovable material extending into the intervertebral foramen (sequestrated annuals, nuclear material, osteophytes). This type of displacement is normally irreducible by physiotherapy.

Adherent nerve root (ANR)

The nerve root becomes shortened and scarred or adhered to its sleeve as a result of trauma or immobility, usually as an initial result of a derangement. Spinal surgery is a common cause of ANR too.

SUBJECTIVE EXAMINATION

All three syndromes usually start with some form of derangement. Sudden onset of spinal pain extending over a few days to the leg. Frequently start for no apparent reason (83%, GGBPS 2007). Most derangements will settle quite quickly but are known to recur. Patients with derangements will often describe numerous episodes of these symptoms over a period of time.

Your subjective examination will have already noted that episodes of back and leg pain are lasting longer and coming on more closely together.

Derangement pain is either constant or intermittent (McKenzie & May 2003).

ANR pain is usually reported as less severe than the original derangement pain.

Pain may be described as being present for several days with increased or constant pain as they continue to carry out normal activities that stretch the nerve root. *After this initial period ANR pain is always intermittent.*

Pain due to entrapment will remain largely the same throughout the history as the compression is always present due to the immobility of the offending material. *Nerve root entrapment pain is constant.*

FACTORS AFFECTING PAIN

Derangement

There will be clear aggravating and easing factors. Flexion activities will increase or peripheralize symptoms. Extended activities will reduce or centralize symptoms. Lying down normally helps.

ANR

Pain is only really produced by positions or activities that stretch the shortened nerve. Sitting is unlikely to be painful, but sitting on the floor will be with legs out in front. Driving often a problem. With ANR an activity that produces leg pain will consistently produce it.

Entrapment

No activity or position will make the pain remain better. Patients generally keep on the move. Most patients describe positions that 'help a little, but soon as that position is released pain returns'.

OBJECTIVE EXAMINATION

In standing posture a *lateral shift* (i.e. shoulders out of alignment when compared with hips/pelvis) is often visible. This is often due to pain and the patient doesn't want to or forgets to put weight on that sore side. In these cases it is correctable. A true shift is much more difficult to correct and more painful, due to a mechanical component.

A lateral shift is *much less likely in ANR* than derangement or entrapment.

If a shift is present in ANR it is most likely as a response to a co-existing derangement.

With ANR deviation in flexion is present, to the same side (ipsilateral) as the pain as the patient tries to avoid over-stretching an already painful and shortened nerve root (a deviation being when the patient does not flex or extend on a sagittal plane but deviates to one side or another).

Deviation in flexion is common in *derangement or entrapment.* This is usually to the opposite side (contralateral) as there is a mechanical block preventing straight flexion. This deviation is generally accompanied by a deviation in extension too. Loss of flexion is very common.

Loss of extension will be present in derangement and entrapment but less common in ANR if underlying derangement.

Table 7.1 gives a summary of these key points.

THE KEY TO DIFFERENTIAL DIAGNOSIS OF REFERRED LEG PAIN

Repeated flexion in standing (FIS) and repeated flexion in lying (FIL).

We are now starting to move deeply into terminology associated with McKenzie Mechanical Diagnosis and Therapy.

However the principles discussed below are related to simple mechanical terminology, which should not handicap you if you have not attended any of these courses but rather suggest simple mechanical and anatomical origins for the patient's leg pain. This will allow you to calm patients and suggest simple effective remedies for reducing their leg pain.

The main identifying feature of entrapment (not from disc but osteophytes) is an increase in range of FIS on repetition as the nerve root is pulled away from the obstruction. *This is not long lasting* and as the patient walks around for a minute the nerve returns to its former limitation.

Table 7.1 Comparison of causes of leg pain referred from lumbar spine

FEATURES	ADHERENT NERVE ROOT	DERANGEMENT	ENTRAPMENT
Pain	Intermittent	Intermittent or constant	Constant
Clinical features	Pain only when shortened structures are stretched – does so CONSISTENTLY	Flexion will increase or peripheralize Extension will decrease or centralize Decreased with lying	No activity/ position will make better
Response to flexion	Flexion in standing will increase or peripheralize Flexion in lying will not produce leg pain	All flexion generally increases leg symptoms	No effect

In a *derangement* FIS will usually increase, worsen or peripheralize the pain. *FIL also will have the same effect.*

With an *ANR*, FIS will also usually increase, worsen or peripheralizes pain. *However FIL will not bring about leg pain as the tension on the nerve root is removed.*

CONCLUSION OF DIFFERENTIAL DIAGNOSIS OF REFERRED LEG PAIN

- Accurate differential diagnosis is important in order to treat patients correctly.
- At worst to stretch and ANR could substantially worsen a misdiagnosed derangement.

- At best, such a derangement would not be reduced. Conversely if ANR is missed the patient will continue to have untreated leg pain.

LUMBAR SPINE PAIN AND PELVIC GIRDLE PAIN

The prevalence of pregnant women suffering from pelvic girdle pain (PGP) is about 20% and although it is possible to focus on and specify PGP, functionally the pelvis cannot be studied in isolation suggesting it is not impossible that there could be separate LBP problem present too (Vleeming et al 2005). See Table 7.2.

Table 7.2 lists some of the key differences in presentation between both pains. As is usually the case the key factor in differential diagnosis of this condition is still a thorough subjective and objective assessment.

Table 7.2 Comparison of lumbar and pelvic pains

FEATURES	LUMBAR PAIN	PELVIC GIRDLE PAIN
Location of pain	Located close to lumbar spine =/l referred symptoms to lower limb(s)	Located more between posterior iliac crest and gluteal fold distal to L5 =/l symphyis pubis pain
		Possibly referred to knee but never calf or foot
Main clinical features	Altered spinal ROM	Full ROM
	Neurological deficits often present	No neurological changes
		'Catching' of the foot
Functional problems	Usually there is some sort of directional preference i.e. specific movement will aggravate or ease symptoms	Worse in sustained positions or movements

The European Guidelines on the Diagnosis and Treatment of Pelvic Girdle Pain (Vleeming et al 2005) have been developed to present the available evidence and to guide treatment of this problem. It is strongly recommended that you have a look at them for one of the most thorough reviews available in this field. The reference section will guide you to the best evidence available.

Similarly any work in this topic area by Diane Lee and Peter O'Sullivan is always the key reference start point when exploring the subject of pelvic control.

Risk factors for developing PGP during pregnancy

- A previous history of LBP
- And/or previous trauma to the pelvis

Non-risk factors

- Time interval since last pregnancy
- Height
- Weight
- Smoking
- Age

SUMMARY OF RECOMMENDATIONS FOR DIFFERENTIAL DIAGNOSIS OF PGP FROM EUROPEAN GUIDELINES

Active straight leg raise test (ASLR)

This has been described as a functional pelvic test. It is recommended that specific attention be paid to pain that comes on during prolonged standing and/or sitting. One way in which you can do this is to ask the patient to either point out the exact location on his/her body, or preferably shade in the painful area on a pain location diagram.

The test is performed with patients in a supine position with legs straight out. The patient is asked to 'try to raise your legs, one after the other, above the couch for 20 cm without bending the knee'.

The patient is asked to score the movement on a 6 point scale:

- Not difficult at all = 0
- Minimally difficult = 1
- Somewhat difficult = 2
- Fairly difficult = 3
- Very difficult = 4
- Unable to do = 5

The scores on both sides are added, so that the sum score range from 0 to 10 (Mens et al 2001). This is then repeated during and after testing.

What do I look for with ASLR?

First, note if there is pain or significant trunk rotation. If the test is negative, add resistance and see if there is pain or trunk rotation.

If either test is positive, try the following and recheck if the test is negative: have the patient actively brace his or her lumbar spine; apply manual compression through the iliac crests; and tighten a belt around the pelvis. Does the pain score change? Does the quality/ease of movement alter?

Clinical consequences of these findings

Pain or poor motor control during ASLR can be caused by SI joint dysfunction or abdominal or hip flexor muscle control problems. A positive test can produce an alteration in load transfer from leg to trunk, and poor pelvic stability during gait or other loading postures or movements (O'Sullivan et al 2002).

GAENSLEN TEST

The patient, lying supine, flexes the knee and hip of the same side, the thigh being crowded against the abdomen with the aid of both the patient's hands clasped about the flexed knee. The patient is then brought well to the side of the table, and the opposite thigh is slowly hyper extended by the examiner with gradually increasing force by pressure of the examiner's hand on the top of the knee. With the opposite hand, the examiner assists the patient in fixing the lumbar spine and pelvis by pressure over the patient's clasped hands. The test is positive if the patient experiences pain, either local or referred on the provoked side (Vleeming et al 2005).

PAIN PROVOCATION OF THE SYMPHYSIS BY MODIFIED TRENDELENBURG'S TEST (STORK TEST)

The patient stands on one leg, flexes the other at 90° in hip and knee. If pain is experienced in the symphysis the test is positive. If the test is positive, try the following and recheck if the test is negative: have the patient actively brace his or her lumbar spine; apply manual compression through the iliac crests; and tighten a belt around the pelvis.

FABER TEST

The subject lies supine. One leg is flexed, abducted, and externally rotated so that the heel rests on the opposite knee. If pain is felt in the SI joints or in the symphysis the test is considered positive (Albert et al 2000).
(Did you know FABER is an abbreviation of Flexion, ABduction and External Rotation??)

POSTERIOR PELVIC PAIN PROVOCATION TEST OR 'THIGH THRUST'

With the patient supine and the hip flexed to 90 degrees on the sore side pressure is applied to the patient's flexed knee along the longitudinal axis of the femur while the pelvis is held steady by the examiner's other hand. The test is positive when the patient feels a familiar well localized pain deep in the gluteal area on the provoked side (Laslett & Williams1994).

SYMPHYSIS PAIN PALPATION TEST

This is perhaps not the best test to carry out without first of all seeking some supervision or guidance from a colleague. With the patient supine, the front side of the pubic symphysis is palpated gently. If any pain is produced that lasts for more than 5 seconds it is recorded as pain. If the pain disappears within 5 seconds it is recorded as tenderness (Albert et al 2000). There is also the conflicting evidence about the poor inter-therapist reliability for palpatory tests.

SPINAL STENOSIS

WHAT IS IT?

Spinal stenosis is a result of degenerative, developmental, or congenital disorders. Spinal stenosis can arise at different areas in the spinal canal, either *central canal stenosis* where bilateral leg pain may occur or in more serious presentations cauda equina syndrome may develop. *Lateral stenosis* may cause more localized nerve root compression (Alvarez & Hardy 1998, Szpalski & Gunzburg 2003).

WHO HAS STENOSIS?

Degenerative stenosis symptoms usually affect men aged more than 50 years. Bilateral symptoms occur with a male:female ratio of 8:1 (Porter 1996).

SYMPTOMS – ONSET

Typically, symptoms are not present at rest.

Usually patients with stenosis complain that symptoms come on walking and standing.

Walking up hill is less painful than walking downhill.

Interestingly Porter (1996) suggests that the walking tolerance (when the patient stops) is usually twice the threshold distance when they first feel discomfort.

SYMPTOMS – EASED

Symptoms are relieved by flexed postures.

When walking, the patient stoops forward, gradually reduces walking speed, and sometimes will stoop forward until he or she finally stops. After a short rest often coping by leaning against a wall, tying a shoe lace or sitting down the patient is able to get going again.

More often than not there are a few neurological changes on objective examination with degenerative stenosis.

‼ CLINICAL CHALLENGE 7.1

Think of how your average degenerative stenotic LBP presents.

What are the other problems that can present? How can these affect both your treatment plans and treatment outcomes?

VASCULAR SYMPTOMS

Symptoms of spinal stenosis are often confused with symptoms associated with vascular claudication such as intermittent claudication. As usual a thorough history taking can help differentiate these differences.

Although a large systematic review of accurate diagnostic clinical tests (with the exception of MRI) is inconclusive (de Graff et al 2006) a nice little test that can aid diagnosis is to ask the patient to try the exercise bike in the department. If leg pains come on in this position it can suggest that there is a larger vascular component. If the patient, *sitting flexed*, can pedal away quite happily working the vascular system but has no leg pain this suggests the possibility for a degenerative stenosis.

PHYSIOTHERAPY FOR DEGENERATIVE STENOSIS

Guess what? Here is no great pile of evidence to provide a successful recipe for the physiotherapy management of stenosis! Think back to Sackett's work. Your evidence based treatment will include the 'Best Available Evidence', 'Your Clinical Experience', and the 'Patient's Expectation'. So use a treatment based on symptom management i.e. don't force extension, use flexion as a friend to cope, pelvic stability, general stamina and strengthening building and refer to orthopaedic and/or imaging if function is worsening.

SACROILIAC JOINT PAIN AND LUMBAR SPINE PAIN

LEAVING THE MOST CONTENTIOUS TO LAST!

The sacroiliac joint (SIJ) as the source of LBP is one of the most heatedly discussed topics I have heard as a clinician. I have seen few topics stir up so much argument among colleagues.

The only thing they can agree upon is that there is no real evidence to back up either camp. This does not mean that some of the world's foremost experts in the treatment of SIJ pain are wrong, because they get many many patients better with their SIJ techniques. Just remember that as a less experienced clinician the more you look for in an LBP assessment the more you will find and in all likelihood the more confused you will get. Before you even start to treat an LBP there are excellent odds that if you got the patient to make and serve the tea in your department for the next four to six weeks their LBP will all but clear up! The whole 'is it LBP or SIJ pain' debate is well worthy of your time and effort. Vleeming's book in the Recommended Reading List is as good a place as any to start.

In writing this book in hopefully a balanced view it is very comfortable sitting on the fence here but if you ever spend some time looking at a cadaveric SIJ you will see that it is:

- One of the strongest joints in the body
- One of the most ligamentous joints in the body
- One of the least flexible joints with very little movement

This alone can lead to doubts about how you would injure it apart from during pregnancy, a traumatic injury or a noticeable onset. Similarly if it is such a strong joint can it be injured in isolation? Repetitive injury due to sustained excessive forces from elsewhere? All food for thought and constructive discussion!

‼ CLINICAL CHALLENGE 7.2

Next time you are on outpatient placement ask your clinical educator what they think of SI joint pain as a reliable source of pain. I would hazard a guess that you will receive one of four answers:

1. Not at all

2. Of course

3. Could be either

4. You are the student/junior. Off you go and reflect and let me know.

These answers will also be more polarized depending on which country you ask them in, reflecting on the general clinical expertise of that area's leading clinicians.

Would you get such ambiguous answers (with the exception of number four, which is the standard clinical educator's response: well one of mine anyway), if you asked 'can lumbar flexion cause LBP?' or 'can an RTA cause whiplash?'?

VALIDITY AND RELIABILITY OF SIJ TESTING

There is a lack of validity and reliability of commonly used clinical SIJ tests often used to plan manual therapy techniques (Van der Wurff et al 1999, 2000). However, difficulties in detecting motion of the SIJ in either symptomatic or asymptomatic individuals challenge the clinical relevance of such findings (Laslett & Williams, 1994, Lee & Vleeming 2000).

Even fluoroscopically guided intra-articular injection or joint block, which are considered the gold standard for diagnosis, still show a false positive rate estimated between 8% and 20% (Laslett et al 2005).

ONE POSSIBLE APPROACH TO HELP IDENTIFY SIJ PROBLEMS

A systematic differential diagnosis approach that has been acknowledged as a useful way of assessing SI/lumbar spine patients has been described by Mark Laslett in a series of articles. (Look at the references and cross referencing in various chapters in the book Vleeming et al edit on the recommended reading list as a starter.)

First of all Laslett & Williams (1994) carried out a review of the reliability of commonly used selected pain provocation tests for SIJ pain. A further study then used these five tests as part of a sub-classification of SIJ and LBP patients (Laslett et al 2003). See Table 7.3.

Laslett started the second part of his work by suggesting that pain originating from the lumbar spine is much more common than specific SI joint pain. He firstly identified patients with suspected lumbar spine pain by carrying out an assessment based on McKenzie's Mechanical Diagnosis and Therapy. Although quite small in numbers this study lays out a nice methodological approach to the differential diagnosis of SI joint pain. Patients who demonstrated peripheralization or centralization (Aina et al 2004) of their symptoms were categorized as having disc problems. Those who had not were then assessed for SIJ problems. If three or more of these SIJ pain provocation tests were positive then a diagnosis of SIJ pain was made.

More recently these diagnostic tests have been further refined and validated. Best evidence now suggests that for symptoms which cannot be centralized the algorithm below should be followed to help in reaching a clearer more structured differential diagnosis. Table 7.3 defines the tests listed in the algorithm in a bit more detail and show how to apply these tests.

Table 7.3 Overview of differential tests Laslett test for SIJ (Laslett & Williams 1994, Laslett et al 2003)

NEW TEST	ACTION	DESIRED EFFECT
Distraction	With your patient supine, you apply a posteriorly directed force to both anterior superior iliac spines	To distract the anterior aspects of the SIJ
Thigh thrust	With the patient supine and the hip flexed to 90 degrees on the sore side pressure is applied to the patient's flexed knee along the longitudinal axis of the femur while the pelvis is held steady by the examiner's other hand (Laslett & Williams 1994, Laslett et al 2003)	To apply a posterior shearing force to the SIJ of that side
Compression test	With your patient lying on one side with hips and knees flexed to about a right angle you apply a vertical force downward on the iliac crest. The shorter of you might be better kneeling on the bed to apply sufficient force	To apply a compression force to both SIJ (Laslett & Williams 1994, Laslett et al 2003)

NEW TEST	**ACTION**	**DESIRED EFFECT**
Sacral thrust 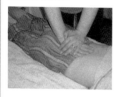	With your patient lying face down you apply a vertical force to the middle of the sacrum	To produce an anterior shearing force of the sacrum on the ilia (Laslett & Williams 1994, Laslett et al 2003)
Gaenslen's test 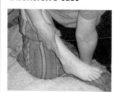	The patient, lying supine, flexes the knee and hip of the same side, the thigh being crowded against the abdomen with the aid of both the patient's hands clasped about the flexed knee. The patient is then brought well to the side of the table, and the opposite thigh is slowly hyper extended by the examiner with gradually increasing force by pressure of the examiner's hand on the top of the knee. With the opposite hand, the examiner assists the patient in fixing the lumbar spine and pelvis by pressure over the patient's clasped hands. (Vleeming et al 2005)	To apply a posterior rotation force to the SIJ on the side of the flexed hip and knee, and an anterior rotation force of the SIJ on the side of the other leg (Laslett & Williams 1994, Laslett et al 2003)

Remember again that the SIJ is a solid structure and you may need to apply more force than you think to reproduce the patient's present symptoms.

Not a quick fix or the only definitive test….but the best evidence we have to date and also a very well thought out, validated, recognized, reproducible and structured starting point to help assess a very complicated clinical condition.

FACET OR ZYGAPOPHYSEAL JOINTS

Revel et al (1992, 1998) have carried out two studies with a similar design to Laslett's work on SIJ, but this time in trying to show when it is more likely the patient's symptoms originate from the facet joints of the lumbar spine. They offer the following list, from which their study estimates that if five out of the seven symptoms are present on examination then the facet joint may be the most likely cause of the patient's pain. Laslett et al (2006) offers an interesting take on further facet joint diagnostic predictors.

- >65 years old
- Pain well relieved by lying down
- No pain coughing
- No pain by forward flexion
- No pain when rising from flexion
- No pain hyperextending
- Pain extension/rotation

However, a word of warning over these tests. It has been suggested that the main bulk of evidence in diagnosing facet joint problems is to carry out a nerve root injection (Laslett et al 2006).

TAKE HOME MESSAGE

Differential diagnosis of lumbar related conditions is very complex and requires a clear thought process, reflection and practice.

Differential diagnosis is not an excuse for jumping to conclusions, but a means to arrive at a more specific diagnosis

that *can help* you plan and execute a more effective treatment for your patients.

Remember differential diagnosis is about using your clinical experience and the literature base to weigh up the probability that one structure more than another is the most likely cause of your patient's symptoms.

Read up on, experiment and test these various differential diagnoses to gain a better understanding of some of your complex LBP patients.

RECOMMENDED READING

Lee D 2004 The Pelvic Girdle. An Approach to the Examination and Treatment of the Lumbopelvic–Hip Region, 3rd edn. Churchill Livingstone, Edinburgh.

Vleeming A, Albert H B, Östgaard H C et al 2005 European guidelines on the diagnosis and treatment of pelvic girdle pain. http://www.backpaineurope.org/web/files/WG4_Guidelines.pdf

Vleeming A, Mooney V, Stoeckart R (eds) 2007 Movement, Stability and Lumbopelvic Pain, 2nd edn. Churchill Livingstone, Edinburgh.

REFERENCES

Aina A, May S, Clare H 2004 The centralisation phenomenon of spinal symptoms: a systematic review. Manual Therapy 9:134-143.

Albert H, Godskesen M, Westergaard J 2000 Evaluation of clinical tests used in classification procedures in pregnancy-related pelvic joint pain. European Spine Journal 9(2):161-166.

Alvarez J A, Hardy R H 1998 Lumbar spine stenosis: a common cause of back and leg pain. American Family Physician 57:1825-1840.

de Graaf L, Prak A, Sita Bierma-Zeinstra S et al 2006 Diagnosis of lumbar spinal stenosis. A systematic review of the accuracy of diagnostic tests. Spine 31(10):1168-1176.

Greater Glasgow Back Pain Service Statistics 2007 (Unpublished).

Klein J G 2005 Five pitfalls in decisions about diagnosis and prescribing. British Medical Journal 330:781-783.

Koriat A, Lichtenstein S, Fischhoff B 1980 Reasons for confidence. Journal of Experimental Psychology: Human Learning & Memory 6:107-118.

Laslett M, Williams M 1994 The reliability of selected pain provocation tests for sacroiliac joint pathology. Spine 19:1243-1249.

Laslett M, Young S B, Aprill C N et al 2003 Diagnosing painful sacroiliac joints: a validity study of a McKenzie evaluation and sacroiliac provocation tests. Australian Journal of Physiotherapy 49:89-97.

Laslett M, Aprill C N, McDonald B et al 2005 Diagnosis of sacroiliac joint pain: validity of individual provocation tests and composites of tests. Manual Therapy 10:207-218.

Laslett M, McDonald B, April C N et al 2006 Clinical predictors of screening lumbar zygapophyseal joint blocks: development of clinical prediction rules. Spine Journal 6(5):370-379.

Lee D, Vleeming A 2000 Diagnostic tools for the impaired pelvis. American Back Society annual meeting, Vancouver.

McKenzie R A, May S 2003 The Lumbar Spine: Mechanical Diagnosis and Therapy (2nd Edn). Spinal Publications, Wellington.

Mens J M A, Vleeming A, Snijders C J et al 2001 Reliability and validity of the active straight leg raise test in posterior pelvic pain since pregnancy. Spine 26(10):1167-1171.

O'Sullivan P B, Beales D J, Beetham J A et al 2002 Altered motor control strategies in subjects with sacroiliac joint pain during the active straight-leg-raise test. Spine 27:EI-E8.

Painting S 1993 The Lumbar Adherent Nerve Root – Differential Diagnosis. McKenzie Newsletter UK 1(2):5-9.

Porter R W 1996 Spinal stenosis and neurogenic claudication. Spine 21(17):2046-2052.

Revel M E, Listrat V M, Chevalier X J 1992 Facet joint block for low back pain: identifying predictors of a good response. Archives of Physical, Medical and Rehabiitation 73:824-828.

Revel M, Poiraudeau S, Auleley G R 1998 Capacity of the clinical picture to characterize low back pain relieved by facet joint anesthesia. Proposed criteria to identify patients with painful facet joints. Spine 23:1972-1977.

Szpalski M, Gunzburg R 2003 Lumbar spinal stenosis in the elderly: an overview. European Spine Journal 12(suppl):170-175.

Vleeming A, Albert HB, Östgaard H C et al 2005 European Guidelines on the Diagnosis and Treatment of Pelvic Girdle Pain. http://www.backpaineurope.org/web/files/WG4_Guidelines.pdf

Van der Wurff P, Meyne W, Hagejier R 1999 Clinical tests of the sacroiliac joint. A systematic methodological review. Part 1: reliability. Manual Therapy 5:30-36.

Van der Wurff P, Meyne W, Hagejier R 2000 Clinical tests of the sacroiliac joint. A systematic methodological review. Part 2: validity. Manual Therapy 5:89–96.

CHAPTER

8

Pain and pharmacology

CONTENTS

IMPORTANT INFORMATION **144**

DEFINITION OF PAIN **144**

WHO HAS PAIN? **145**

HOW DOES PAIN GO AWAY? **146**

DIMENSIONS OF PAIN **147**

ADAPTIVE AND MALADAPTIVE PAIN **149**

PAIN MECHANISMS **151**

PHARMACOLOGICAL MANAGEMENT **153**

AIMS AND OBJECTIVES

Aim: To introduce the concept of pain and the different types of pain and the effect of the correct medication on them for patients with LBP

Objectives: By the end of the chapter the reader will be able to:

1. Identify the different types of pain
2. Discuss the different presentations of different types of pain
3. Identify the correct medication for different types of pain

IMPORTANT INFORMATION

This chapter is a brief overview of pain and the early pharmacological management in the assessment of patients with symptoms associated with LBP.

Although this chapter discusses LBP (meaning lumbar pain and/or leg pain) the information should be seen as transferable to all patients you see who are in pain.

The information to follow will help you achieve the aim and objectives of the chapter. And in turn to become more aware of the complex issue that pain is and how this awareness can have positive effects on your LBP assessments.

This chapter is not an in-depth text on pain. As you will probably know the area of pain is a vast, complex and challenging one. Your knowledge and your patients' welfare will be served further by having a look at the additional resources listed below.

I warmly acknowledge my colleague Ellen Daly who I have listened to many times speak so knowledgably about this topic. Some of it must have filtered through.

RECOMMENDED ADDITIONAL RESOURCES ON THE TOPIC OF PAIN

Butler & Moseley 2003 Explain Pain. ISBN 0-9750910-0-X. NOI Group Publications, Adelaide.

Topical issues in pain (www.achesandpainsonline.com).

Pain master classes are run by the Greater Glasgow Back Pain Service (www.nhsggc.org.uk/ggbps) in conjunction with the Physiotherapy Pain Association (North) (www.ppaonline.org.uk).

A DEFINITION OF PAIN: ACUTE AND CHRONIC

It is unlikely there is consensus of just one definition of pain. The International Association for the Study of Pain (IASP 1986) has defined pain *as an unpleasant sensory and emotional experience associated with actual or potential tissue damage, or described in terms of such damage*.

From a patient's point of view *'pain is whatever the experiencing person says it is, existing when he/she says it does'* (McCaffery & Pasero 1999). Acute pain generally has a biological function–it warns the patient over damage or possible damage to body tissues (Melzack & Wall 1996). Acute pain has usually cleared up before healing is complete between a few days to a few weeks (Loesar & Melzack 1999).

Acute pain is perhaps most eloquently described by Melzack & Wall (1998) who suggest that acute pain *'offers the hope of future recovery'*.

…………this perceived lack of hope is a more common feature of chronic pain.

Pain, which persists after the expected time for normal tissue healing has passed or where healing does not take place, has been defined by one of the leading forums in the field as chronic pain (IASP 1986). As Chapter 4 discussed, chronic pain may be accompanied by severe psychological and social disturbance.

The Pain in Europe Survey (2003) has suggested that pain of less than 3 months is acute pain and pain present for over 3–6 months is chronic pain.

‼ CLINICAL CHALLENGE 8.1

On your next clinical day…….how many patients did you treat that day who had no pain?

WHO HAS PAIN?

The easiest clinical challenge to answer to date! (although probably the most complex to deal with!).

Is it just musculoskeletal physiotherapists who deal with pain? *Of course not!*

Pain is present in orthopaedic patients, ICU patients, Care of the Elderly, Paediatrics, Medical or Stroke Units, Mental Health, Obstetrics and Gynaecology etc……

The Pain in Europe Report (2003) doesn't really paint the happiest picture of pain:

- In Europe chronic pain strikes one in five adults.
- Back pain is the most common site of pain reported by chronic pain sufferers (24%).
- One-third of patients suffer chronic pain at all times.
- People with chronic pain have had their symptoms for an average of 7 years.

Does this sound a familiar presentation in many of your patients????

HOW DOES PAIN GO AWAY?

Generally the first thing an LBP patient asks is 'when will the pain go?'.

Why else have the majority of these patients bothered to self refer or see their GP for a physiotherapy referral.........they are in pain.

We would all love pain when present to just go. Just like that! (See Figure 8.1). How easy it would be to show patients the graph they want to see. In 'x-amount' of days you will be pain free.

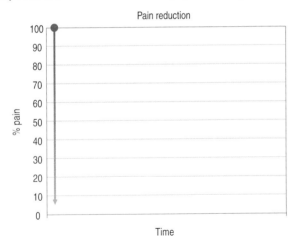

FIG 8.1 How we would all like pain to go?

Unfortunately, if and when pain goes it actually tends to go as shown in Figure 8.2. It is a gradual thing. Note the much longer 'Time' axis here. With no definitive timescale. Often there are days when the pain 'flares up' for no reason. 'I don't know what did, but things were doing great until yesterday. It's so frustrating.'

This is an all too common, and justified, complaint from patients.

'What I think has done me the world of good in all honesty' (patient quote from Rose, in Gifford 1997) Medicalization of pain?

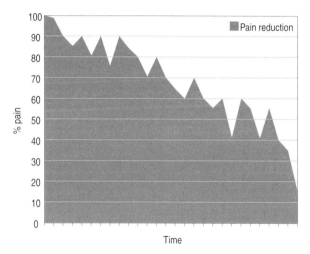

FIG 8.2 How pain normally goes.

Just explaining how pain normally goes to patients can have excellent results in helping patients understand their pain (Butler & Gifford 2003). If nothing else, doing this can begin to calm the anxious patient and perhaps go some way to addressing possible yellow flags.

DIMENSIONS OF PAIN

From what we have seen so far it is clear that pain is multi-dimensional. So then, should our treatment not be too? Butler & Gifford (1998) explain in excellent detail the three dimensions of pain.

What Butler and Gifford are getting at is to look at your patient with LBP from more than one side. Yes the sensory dimension will cause the patient discomfort and loss of sleep and will heal in 6–8 weeks.........but this is affected for good or bad by thoughts and emotions.

N.B. As a rule of thumb anything written on pain by David Butler and Louis Gifford is always worth reading to improve your knowledge of pain.

SENSORY

This is the dimension that most of our physical assessment focuses on. It's one of the reasons we fill in a body chart, when we ask about:

- Where is your LBP?   (Site)
- How sore is the pain?   (Intensity)
- How would you describe your LBP?   (Quality and type)

COGNITIVE

This dimension refers to how patients use coping strategies either helpful or unhelpful to their benefit or detriment. It links with the information in Chapter 4 about A, B, C, D, E, F and W of yellow flags.

- What are your previous experiences of LBP?
- How is your LBP affecting your lifestyle?
- What do you think is the cause of your LBP?
- What can you do to make your LBP go away?

EMOTIONAL

This dimension, with the individual responses to the cognitive dimension, dictate how the patient behaves in relation to their LBP.

- Fear
- Anger
- Worry etc......

Again, look over the yellow flags chapter to tie this together.

ADAPTIVE AND MALADAPTIVE PAIN

How a patient copes with their LBP, either through useful or less useful behaviour, is their attempt to resolve their problem (Turk et al 2001).

Adaptive pain can be seen as being useful to help create the optimal environment to allow recovery of normal function and healing, for example, a patient with acute LBP who gets relief by walking about rather than sitting. The sustained flexing of the lumbar spine while sitting is causing the pain.

Maladaptive pain on the other hand is when there is no obvious pathological reason for the LBP. The pain itself is now the problem. Pain is now the disease, pain is now maladaptive, or of no use at all (Gifford 1997).

CASE STUDY 8.1

John is 55 years old. He had his first episode of LBP and pain in S1 area of his left lower limb 3 years ago. Symptoms have never gone away since. He 'just gets on with it'. Recently his daughter has encouraged John to attend physiotherapy 'as symptoms are not going away'. He has no red flags apart from his age and pain on coughing. His physiotherapy records from 3 years ago show he had reduced ankle jerk reflex, S1 myotome loss and straight leg raise reduced to 20 degree on the left and painful. Last week on first assessment, the only neurological change still present was reduced straight leg raise. John is very proud that he has never had a day off work as a postman in over two years. Lumbar flexion was markedly reduced. John walks with a limp and his left hip is noticeably externally rotated. When questioned about the need to correct his altered gait pattern, John replied 'this is the only way I can walk about with reduced pain. What will happen if I change it now?'

Compare this to Bob. He has an identical initial presentation. However, his leg pain was abolished within four weeks. Bob also has an altered gait pattern. His left hip is externally rotated and he keeps his back very

---

(Continued)

straight. Bob though feels that because of his ongoing, intermittent central LBP, he isn't quite ready for work. He has been avoiding any lifting because when he does bend forward he has 'pain in the middle of his back'.

QUESTIONS ON CASE STUDY 8.1

It would be fair to say that John and Bob have maladaptive pain.

Q1.

Is maladaptive pain always harmful?

Q2.

How can you justify John's altered gait pattern?

Q3.

Can maladaptive pain ever be useful? Is it useful in Bob's instance?

It is unlikely there really is a definitive answer to these questions, especially question two, but it is perhaps thinking of the three dimensions of pain that can help to make more sense of this.

‼ CLINICAL CHALLENGE 8.2

This is a textbook on LBP (hopefully you will have noticed by now!).

Pain should though be considered by ALL physiotherapists.

Consider if there was adaptive or maladaptive pain present the next time you deal with a patient on an acute surgical ward, or an Intensive Care Unit or a paediatric neurological outpatient clinic.

The challenge of pain is everywhere. Are physiotherapists provided with enough training to deal with this everyday, complex issue? (See important information at the start of this chapter for help.)

PAIN MECHANISMS

Pain mechanisms describe the pathobiology of pain. For the purpose of this text they can be classified into three areas.

NOCICEPTIVE PAIN

This is pain originating from damaged tissues such as muscles, tendons, joints, bones as a result of nerves being stimulated in them.

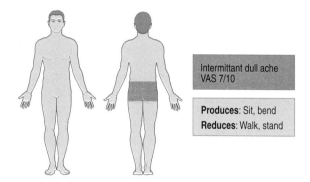

Intermittant dull ache
VAS 7/10

Produces: Sit, bend
Reduces: Walk, stand

FIG 8.3 Nociceptive pain.

A common presentation is shown in the body in Figure 8.3. Look at the words used by the patient to describe their symptoms. This pain is usually as a result of an acute injury with an obvious pathology, e.g. a soft-tissue injury somewhere in the lumbar spine due to a heavy lift with a sudden onset of central LBP.

PERIPHERAL NEUROGENIC PAIN

This is pain generated from within the nervous system from the nerve root, nerve trunk or nervi nervorum (nerves distributed to the sheaths of nerve trunks). A common presentation is shown in the body in Figure 8.4. Look at segmental presentation of the leg pain and how the pain is described.

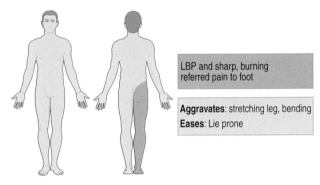

LBP and sharp, burning referred pain to foot

Aggravates: stretching leg, bending
Eases: Lie prone

FIG 8.4 Peripheral neurogenic pain.

Patients with peripheral neurogenic LBP tend to present with lower limb symptoms in a dermatomal and/or myotomal distribution (Hall & Elvey 1999). These neurogenic symptoms are very often described as sharp, shooting, hot or burning (Jackson 2006), e.g. nerve root pain.

Central neurogenic. In this situation pain is produced as the result of impulses being generated from within the central nervous system that are interpreted as pain. This can be from dorsal horn cells to the whole brain.

A common presentation is shown in the body in Figure 8.5. Look at the more unusual and stranger presentation of this patient.

SYMPATHETIC/MOTOR

This is pain as a result of activity in the autonomic or motor systems. The resultant pain is thought to be due to the secretions of nociceptor sensitizing chemicals, which cause

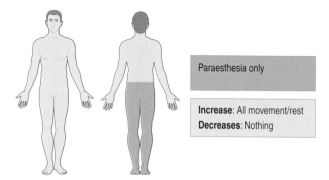

Paraesthesia only

Increase: All movement/rest
Decreases: Nothing

FIG 8.5 Central neurogenic pain.

nerve terminals or injured axons to fire and cause pain, e.g. repetitive strain injury or complex regional pain syndrome.

AFFECTIVE

This is pain produced as a result of emotional and cognitive influences, such as anxiety, fear or anger.

PHARMACOLOGICAL MANAGEMENT

'The drugs don't work they just make you worse..........'

'.........In America in 2000 44 million prescriptions were written for 24.5 million patients with LBP both acute and chronic.' (Luo et al 2004)

Never assume that because a patient has seen their GP that they have been prescribed the correct medication. Equally never assume that because a patient has been prescribed a list of drugs that they are (*a*) *taking them at all or* (*b*) *taking them as prescribed.*

It has been regularly suggested that patients do not always take their medication as prescribed. An estimate that about 6–20% of patients fail even to redeem their prescriptions and 30–50% delay or omit doses (Giuffrida & Torgerson 1997) should set off alarm bells. This should be your starting point: *'Are you taking your medication as prescribed?'*

Box 8.1   IMPORTANT INFORMATION

This section does not suggest that physiotherapists start giving advice, prescribe medication, alter doses etc. That is an argument for another day!

Each Health Board, Primary Care Trust and physiotherapy department will have their own policies and procedures for what advice can be given to patients.

The following information is to enable the reader to have a basic understanding of what is recommended as the best medication for the appropriate condition.

The information in this section will enable you, confidently and with evidence backed argument, to challenge and discuss alternatives to the patient's present medication with their GP. You will also be able to reassure and support patients on the pain management.

Incidentally I have never known a GP not to review a patient's medication on a suggestion from physiotherapists.

WORLD HEALTH ORGANIZATION (WHO) ANALGESIA LADDER

The WHO analgesia ladder was developed to guide prescribers in the graded use of medication (WHO 1986).

Choice of medication is directed by the severity, the type and cause of the pain. Type, cause and severity can only be determined from a thorough patient assessment (SIGN 2000). (See Fig. 8.6 for a diagrammatic representation of this.)

DRUG THERAPY

NHS Greater Glasgow and Clyde Pain Resource Manual, 2002 (with permission).

Nociceptive pain

- Non-opioid analgesics
  - Use at regular intervals
  - 1st line – Paracetamol

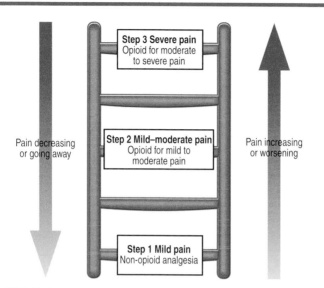

FIG 8.6 World Health Organization Analgesic Ladder (World Health Organization, 1986).

- 2nd line – NSAIDs
- Muscle relaxants
  - Short term – 1 week max
  - e.g. Diazepam, baclofen

Neuropathic/neurogenic pain

- Opioids – tricyclic antidepressants
  - Simple analgesics not as helpful
  - NSAIDs not always helpful

e.g. Amitriptyline, gabapentin or pregabalin helpful as first-stage management.

Tricyclic antidepressants

'Opioids are amongst the most powerful analgesics but politics, prejudice and continuing ignorance impede optimum prescribing.......patients with chronic pain may suffer longer and unnecessarily if we prescribe and legislate badly.' (McQuay 2001)

> ## ‼ CLINICAL CHALLENGE 8.3
>
> Although McQuay's quotation was in respect of pain control in cancer patients it hints at a strong belief that opioids are beneficial to patients with peripheral neurogenic pain.
>
> Why do you think the problems listed above are there?
>
> What, if anything, can physiotherapists do about some or all of them?
>
> This should get you thinking! This won't be a quick challenge…it may take you many years to improve pain control in the area you work…however an understanding of the problems and possible solutions will help you in the short and longer term.

WORDS OF CAUTION ABOUT SUGGESTING A PATIENT SEE THEIR GP ABOUT THEIR SUITABILITY FOR TRICYCLIC ANTIDEPRESSANTS

These medications are normally best taken 12 hours before a patient expects to normally get up the next morning. This allows for maximum benefit on the neurogenic pain with minimal drowsiness side effects. Amitriptyline is the most commonly prescribed such medication I have seen given for this sort of pain. Amitriptyline, in much higher doses, is commonly used to treat depression.

Often a GP may not have time to explain this fully to an already distressed patient, who then gets a prescription with 'antidepressant' blazoned across the box! They quite regularly don't take it or lose confidence in the therapist who thinks the pain is all in their mind. Taking a bit of time to set out the whole situation to the patient, before you ask their GP to consider amitriptyline is well worth it. Explain the pain and explain the medication……you are not prescribing……just using your knowledge to advise the patient on the facts.

Also an amitriptyline dose normally starts low at around 10 mg and increases gradually in 10 mg or 25 mg increments. Full benefit is often not achieved for up to 4 weeks. If your patient has neurogenic pains consider these parameters before changing your mind.

Physiotherapists are prime managers of pain, often more skilled in this very specialized area than many GPs or other health care professionals. We are not telling them their job… just guiding them on the best evidence based pathway.

Think back to the red flag and yellow flag chapters. Be confident in your clinical reasoning and reflective skills; you are consistently reviewing any possible dangerous red flags and helping to give a consistent message to your patient.

Leeds Assessment of Neuropathic Symptoms and Signs pain scale (S-LANSS) is a validated tool for assessing the presence of neuropathic pain (Bennett et al 2005). Easy to administer to patients when you are not too sure about their pain. Check this out via the following link: www.neurocentre.com/slanss.pdf.

This is really just the tip of the metaphorical pain iceberg. Pain mechanisms and neurophysiology are all extremely complex topics but equally exciting areas. If every patient you see has some degree of pain then are we not morally and professionally obliged as health care professionals to learn as much about these areas as possible rather than just go on manual therapy based courses alone?

Fortunately we are at a time and place where pain is starting to be understood and explained to clinicians as well as patients. Instead of letting your heart sink at another patient with pain go out and read Mosley's and Gifford's work. Bother your managers until they allow you to buy *Topical Issues on Pain* and other fine pain works!

TAKE HOME MESSAGE

Pain can and normally does affect every patient you assess and treat as a physiotherapist.

The pain problem is not exclusive to the patients but family, friends, partners, colleagues can all be affected.

Explaining pain to patients and friends can reassure them all about a very distressing situation. This can have positive effects on the outcome of your physiotherapy treatment.

The correct medication, at the correct time for the correct pain is the correct option!

ADDITIONAL READING/INFORMATION

Butler and Moseley 2003 Explain Pain. ISBN 0-9750910-0-X, NOI Group Publications, Adelaide.

Topical issues in pain (www.achesandpainsonline.com).

Anything by Louis Gifford or Lorimar Moseley.

REFERENCES

Bennett M I, Smith B H, Torrance N et al 2005 The S-LANSS score for identifying pain of predominantly neuropathic origin: validation for use in clinical and postal research. Journal of Pain 6(3):149-158.

Butler D S, Gifford L 1998 The Dynamic Nervous System. NOI Press, Adelaide.

Butler D, Moseley L 2003 Explain Pain. NO1 Group Publications, Adelaide.

Gifford L 1997 Pain. In: Pitt-Brooke J, Reid H, Lockwood J et al (eds) Rehabilitations of Movement. WB Saunders, Philadelphia.

Gifford L, Butler D 1997 Integration of the pain sciences into clinical practise. Journal of Hand Therapy 10:86-95.

Giuffrida A, Torgerson D J 1997 Should we pay the patient? Review of financial incentives to enhance patient compliance. BMJ 315: 703-707.

Greater Glasgow and Clyde Pain Resource Manual 2002 Unpublished.

Hall T, Elvey B 1999 Nerve trunk pain: physical diagnosis and treatment. Manual Therapy 4(2):63-73.

International Association for the Study of Pain 1986 Classification of chronic pain. Pain (suppl) 3:S1-S226.

Jackson K D 2006 Pharmacotherapy for neuropathic pain. Pain Practice 6(1):27-33.

Luo X, Pietrobon R et al 2004 Prescription of nonsteroidal anti-inflammatory drugs and muscle relaxants for back pain in the United States. Spine 29:E531-E537.

McCaffery M, Pasero C 1999 Clinical Management. Mosby, St Louis.

McQuay H 2001 Opioids in chronic non-malignant pain. BMJ 322: 1134-1135.

Melzack R, Wall P D 1996 The Challenge of Pain, 2nd edn. Penguin Books, London.

Loeser J D, Melzack R 1999 Pain: an overview. Lancet 353:1607-1609.

Pain in Europe A 2003 Report. Janet Fricker in association with Mundipharma International. Cambridge 2003.

Scottish Inter Collegiate Network (SIGN) 2000 Guideline no 44 Control of pain in patients with cancer. www.sign.ac.uk

Turk D, Melzak R in Okifuji A, Anders K, Cleeland C 2001 Handbook of pain assessment, 2nd edn. Guilford Press, England.

World Health Organization 1986 Analgesic Ladder www.who.int/cancer/palliative/painladder.

Physiotherapy treatments for LBP: clinical guidelines and the importance of evidence-based medicine

CHAPTER

9

CONTENTS

INTRODUCTION 162

TRADITIONAL PHYSIOTHERAPY
TREATMENTS FOR LBP 162

PHYSIOTHERAPY CONSENSUS
ON LBP INTERVENTIONS 167

TREATMENTS ACTUALLY GIVEN
BY UK PHYSIOTHERAPISTS 168

GUIDANCE AND SUPPORT ON
MANAGEMENT OF LBP 169

EVIDENCE-BASED MEDICINE 185

AIMS AND OBJECTIVES

Aims:
1. To have knowledge of the clinical effectiveness of the physiotherapy treatments commonly used to treat LBP
2. To have an understanding of the components of evidence-based medicine
3. To be aware and understand the relevance of the most recent guidelines for the clinical management of acute low back pain, especially those related to the United Kingdom

Objectives: At the end of this chapter you should be able to:
1. Discuss the clinical effectiveness of commonly used physiotherapy treatments for LBP
2. Demonstrate an understanding of why guidelines are used
3. Be aware of the relevant and most recent clinical guidelines for LBP
4. Identify the concepts of evidence-based medicine
5. Identify areas in your clinical practice that require work to allow you to begin to practice in an evidence-based manner
6. Incorporate these practices into your day-to-day management of LBP

INTRODUCTION

Previous chapters (if you are still awake?) have already shown you:
1. What a problem LBP is
2. The importance of assessing for RED FLAGS, YELLOW FLAGS and CES
3. How to carry out a thorough, safe and useful subjective and objective examination
4. How to move towards differential diagnosis of LBP patients
5. About differing types of pain mechanisms and pain management

The remaining chapters will focus more on how you could, how you should, and how others already have managed LBP, based on clinical guidelines, evidence-based medicine and, in some cases, innovative practice.

Although we are highly skilled clinicians (never doubt your own worth) physiotherapy management of LBP is based upon you offering what we think of as the best treatment for our individual patients supported by clinical guidelines in an attempt to practice some sort of evidence-based medicine.

TRADITIONALLY USED PHYSIOTHERAPY TREATMENTS FOR LBP

The treatments offered by physiotherapists for patients with LBP can really be boiled down to two different categories: passive treatments or active treatments.

Passive interventions include, heat, cold, mobilization, manipulation, massage, corset use, traction, electrical stimulation, or acupuncture (Foster et al 1999, van Tulder et al 1997, 2000).

Active treatments include non-specific exercise (Foster et al 1999, van Tulder et al 2000), specific exercises (Long et al 2004) or some forms of manual therapy, for example mechanical diagnosis and therapy (McKenzie 2005).

Over the last two decades there have been OVER 1000 randomized control trials and systematic reviews of the traditionally practised physiotherapy interventions for LBP. (Have you read them all yet? Are you going to add to it soon? Also bear in mind that is only the number of RCTs and does not include the many more non-randomized and controlled trials carried out!)

There has been a consistent agreement that comparison between these studies is difficult. One of the main reasons is that there is a lack of a standard agreed definition for 'low back pain'. This can make actual direct comparisons between treatments difficult (Frost et al 2004, Pengel et al 2003, van Tulder et al 2000, 2004a, b, Waddell et al 1998). Similarly, the ongoing issue of no standardized classification system for LBP is an issue. Table 9.1 highlights some of the evidence presented with respect to systematic reviews of general management of LBP.

These wide ranging systematic reviews have been listed in the Cochrane Database, which has been consistently recognized as among the best quality systematic reviews in medical research (Jadad et al 2000, Oxman & Guyatt 1991).

The biomedical model, so evident in the past in the NHS, focuses on the physical processes, such as the pathology and the physiology of a condition in comparison to the biopsychosocial model encompassing biological, psychological and social factors (Engel 1977, Turk & Flor 1984). The physiotherapy management of patients today indicates that the biopsychosocial model is becoming common practice among physiotherapists (Chou 2005, Daykin & Richardson 2004, Ostelo et al 2003).

We don't really know what the best treatment for LBP is.

If you explore clinical guidelines and published papers the evidence hints at an active treatment that encourages a return to normal function as soon as possible with a patient provided with quality evidence on their condition; namely the *Back Book*.

- After that……well……who knows……

Whatever treatment you offer your patients a good starting point should always be 'what physiological changes is my treatment offering?'.

- Is my manual therapy technique actually having a physiological effect on that 'prolapsed disc?'
- 'If a patient's LBP shoots down their leg when they flex in standing or lying…….why am I getting them to extend?'

Table 9.1 Cochrane review of LBP treatments

INTERVENTION	AUTHOR/YEAR OF RECENT UPDATE	COCHRANE REVIEW	AUTHORS' CONCLUSIONS
Bed rest/advice to stay active	Hagen et al (2004)	Increased pain levels and poorer function with bed rest compared to staying active. No difference for sciatica patients between bed rest and staying active. Evidence to recommend staying active including work	Evidence remains strong for avoiding bed rest and keeping active. Studies of sufficient quality
Psychosocial risk factors	Karjalainen et al (2003)	Assess psychosocial risk factors early and review if there is no improvement in overall condition	Some benefits shown but lack of cost effectiveness in outcomes reduces impact
Surgery for disc prolapse	Gibson & Waddell (2006)	Strong evidence that sciatica patients have faster relief of pain than with conservative management. Long-term effect unknown	Only 3 studies directly compared surgical versus non-surgical patients. Evidence would suggest surgery for sciatic pain on specially selected patients is beneficial. However, due to potential for bias and lack of listed complications review should be read with caution

Table 9.1 Cont'd

INTERVENTION	AUTHOR/YEAR OF RECENT UPDATE	COCHRANE REVIEW	AUTHORS' CONCLUSIONS
Manipulation	Assendelft et al (2003)	Manipulation superior to sham treatment for short term benefit but no difference compared to GP care, analgesia, exercises	39 randomized control trials were found. Definition of back pain population makes direct comparison between studies difficult
Exercise therapy	Hayden et al (2005)	Review to Feb 2000. No difference between exercise therapy, inactive or other active treatments	Results should be treated with some caution due to low quality studies with poor outcome measures and inconsistent and poor reporting
Acupuncture	Furlan et al (2006)	Reviewed to Feb 2003. No conclusions possible in acute low back pain	3 randomized control trials with low participant numbers and poor methodology
Transcutaneous nerve stimulation (TENS)	Khadilkar et al (2005)	Not recommended for acute LBP	Insufficient evidence as only 2 randomized control trials; showing more effective than paracetamol

These examples do not necessarily show that these particular treatments are wrong. You need to be able though to honestly reflect on what physiological changes you are AIMING for with a certain treatment and what ACTUAL physiological changes you have brought about…if any. Or is it just your gentle touch and caring nature that have produced a reduction in pain?

Arrange an in-service at your local anatomy lab. Look at the anatomy of the spine and think about what your normal treatments are actually doing to the tissues.

‼ CLINICAL CHALLENGE 9.1

Think of your last two LBP patients.

Put aside research and clinical guidelines……

What actual physiological changes did you impact on their spine as a result? (Be honest.)

Could you justify these changes to an anatomist or physiologist?

‼ CLINICAL CHALLENGE 9.2

Look at some of the treatments for LBP reviewed by Cochrane Group (Table 9.1).

1. Which treatments listed here have you used to treat LBP patients? Did they get better with it?

2. Have you ever used some of the treatments 'not recom-mended' by the Cochrane Group? Did the patient get better anyway with you giving that treatment 'with little evidence'? If they did, does that mean you are right and Cochrane are wrong? Should you stop giving these 'not recommended treatments'? Does this mean you are living life on the edge and treating patients in an 'non-evidence-based fashion'? (See Evidence Based information a bit later.)

3. Do you think the treatments you offer for LBP today will be same in 3 years/6 years/10 years? Why?

Look at the potential confusion around spinal manipulation for LBP. Two very large and authoritative studies have produced conflicting conclusions around the usefulness of this particular treatment for LBP. Assendelt et al study published in 2003 found no evidence for the effectiveness of manipulation for LBP, following a review of 39 randomized control studies. This was a large Cochrane based review carrying significant kudos in the academic world. However, the more recently published BEAM study (UK BEAM 2004) found manipulation with or without exercises improved symptoms more than 'best care' alone. This study was awarded significant amounts of financial support and was carried out in different areas throughout the UK. It has since been published as a model of good practice.

- *Is it simply a case of right and wrong?*

It is more likely a case of different client groups and different inclusion criteria for studies to be reviewed. This is a grey area, where you could be right or wrong in administering this treatment. It is all part of weighing up the evidence. (See Evidence Based Section a bit later.) Also sometimes you need to examine the studies in a more critical way rather than just reading the conclusion! In these two studies the respondents in the BEAM trial were osteopaths, chiropractors and manipulative physiotherapists who worked in NHS and in private practice thereby differing significantly from the expert physiotherapy panel in the current study. This could explain the different opinions with respect to manipulation being used to manage LBP. It could also be suggested that the perceived level of skill and confidence in manipulation felt by the respondents may be a factor.

While there is little strong evidence to specify one particular physiotherapy treatment over another that does not necessarily mean nothing we do is useful to help LBP patients (or at least I hope not or there isn't much point in writing and reading further!). Our best input is to weigh up the evidence with other factors (see a bit further below).

PHYSIOTHERAPY CONSENSUS ON LBP INTERVENTIONS

A few studies have made attempts to look at the physiotherapy treatment from another angle by investigating levels of physiotherapists' consensus in the management of LBP (Battie et al 1994, Foster et al 1999, Gracey et al 2001, Li & Bombardier 2001, Mikhail et al 2005).

All of these studies (Battie et al 1994, Foster et al 1999, Gracey et al 2001, Li & Bombardier 2001, Mikhail et al 2005) propose the physiotherapy interventions for the management of LBP have changed in the last decade from a biomedical model to a more biopsychosocial model of care………a good thing?

Mikhail et al (2005) found in 68% of their study sample there was the prevalence of use of interventions with strong or moderate evidence of effectiveness. However over 90% of the therapists' surveyed still used interventions for which research evidence was limited or absent. Those therapists who used more evidence-based interventions were more recently qualified and had attended more postgraduate courses than the non-users. (Namely, the group who are specifically targeted by this book. Ready for the challenge??)

WHAT TREATMENTS PHYSIOTHERAPISTS IN THE UK ACTUALLY GIVE

I imagine there have been many local studies and audits investigating what treatments physiotherapists give to their LBP patients. (If you have been involved in one then let people know. No point keeping all your good work secret. There is no reason this information cannot contribute to the ongoing debate.)

Two of the most influential published studies in the UK have asked physiotherapists what treatments they give to patients with LBP. Foster et al (1999) found a preference among physiotherapists for manual therapy for the treatment of LBP. Forty eight percent of the respondents reported that they commonly used electrotherapy treatments. While not investigating this use further, the fact so many respondents even had a preference could lead to the suggestion the use of electrotherapy is still very common in the treatment of LBP.

Gracey et al (2001) highlight the use of advice as being given in almost 90% of patients. This is in line with most of the current evidence (Hay et al 2005), which has reported on the benefits of advice being given as part of a pain management programme. The study results though do not expand further on the actual form and type of advice given. The advice given could have been 'don't walk down stairs when you have your hands in your pocket,' so we cannot be sure exactly if a consistent and effective message is given to patients.

A more recent study suggested that an expert panel of physiotherapy clinicians can reach consensus on the physiotherapy management of LBP, and that this consensus sits in line with the evidence base (Ferguson et al 2008). An omission from this study is that it did not explore if these good intentions were actually carried over into clinical practice….yet!

The Back Book (www.tsoshop.co.uk) is the only piece of patient education that has proved effective in an RCT (Burton et al 1999).

WHERE CAN I GO FOR GUIDANCE AND SUPPORT TO MANAGE LBP PATIENTS THEN: A QUICK GUIDE TO CLINICAL GUIDELINES

WHAT ARE CLINICAL GUIDELINES?

As physiotherapists managing LBP we have been supplied with clinical guideline after clinical guideline. Often it looks like (or we hope in anticipation that it is) each guideline is a means to a better life for the concerned physiotherapist and the generally anxious patient. In theory these benefits should not just be restricted to one professional but in theory should assist physiotherapists, GPs, orthopaedic surgeons and imagers too, in planning a similar approach to the management of this major health and social problem.

Clinical guidelines however, have been defined as systematically developed statements designed to *help* practitioners and patients *decide* on the most *appropriate and effective* healthcare for specific clinical conditions (Field & Lohr 1992).

These guidelines have been developed as the result of systematic reviews and bring together the *best available clinical evidence*, which has been the product of expert consensus (Borkan & Cherkin 1996, Deyo & Phillips 1996, van Tulder et al 1997, 2000).

Word of caution……clinical guidelines do not offer a secret cure to the management of LBP!!

Clinical guidelines are based on the best available high quality evidence and are comparable with current evidence-based practices (Grimmer et al 2003, Shekelle at al 1999).

Clinical guidelines have relevance to your clinical practice no matter where you work. For example, where I practice within Scotland, recent political and professional pressures have insisted the management of LBP must be clinically effective, and ineffective treatments have been rooted out (CSP 2004, Scottish Executive 2003, 2005, Scottish Office 1998).

HOW TO SUCCESSFULLY DEVELOP CLINICAL GUIDELINES?

The most successfully implemented clinical guidelines are those developed in partnership between expert and grass roots input, a balance between recognized world experts and researchers in the field of LBP and researchers/clinicians and physiotherapists who manage LBP on a day-to-day basis.

One way in which to improve the increase of evidence-based physiotherapy intervention is by the dissemination and implementation of this evidence base to all therapists managing LBP (Mikhail et al 2005).

Too little grassroots ownership may result in an erosion of professional autonomy (Grimmer et al 2003, Moore & Jull 2003). On the other hand, if too much local input is credited with the development of guidelines this may result in a reduction in credibility of guidelines, with possible problems with acceptance and implementation: yet another delicate balancing act!

EFFECTIVENESS OF CLINICAL GUIDELINES

Some studies have attempted to assess the impact of these RCGP guidelines in the UK by investigating GP, consultant and nursing opinions (Barnett et al 1999, Dey et al 2004) with varying success. However for the vast financial sums of money spent in

> **CLINICAL CHALLENGE 9.3**
>
> Does the department you work in at the moment have any of their own clinical guidelines?
>
> If so dust them down and compare them to those listed in Table 9.2.
>
> Are there any great areas of consensus?
>
> How could your department's guidelines be improved?

their development the evidence base on their effectiveness is disappointing.

The most common problems affecting the successful impact of clinical guidelines are (Barnett et al 1999, Dey et al 2004):

- Involvement in guideline development
- Dissemination of guidelines
- Lack of help in their implementation

It could be suggested that an additional more common problem that really affects the successful impact of clinical guidelines: THERE ARE JUST TOO MANY OF THEM! The vast number of these guidelines can lead to many problems with confusion over which to follow as just a starting point!

CLINICAL GUIDELINES WORTHWHILE AND ADHERED TO?

There have been no large studies published which have attempted to show if physiotherapists actually adhere to clinical guidelines anyhow. So while empirical evidence would suggest that clinical guidelines are beneficial to patients, we do not know if physiotherapists actually bother to follow them…yet.

> **CLINICAL CHALLENGE 9.4**
>
> What do you think are three of the main benefits of clinical guidelines for LBP?

At the time of writing this book, Quality Improvement Scotland are about to begin a NATIONAL PHYSIOTHERAPY LOW BACK PAIN AUDIT. If you explore their web site, www.nhshealthquality. org/nhsqis/4057.html, you should be able to see the final results, which are due to be published in March 2009, with interim results available in July/August 2008. As far as I am aware this will be the first project of its kind.

‼ CLINICAL CHALLENGE 9.5

If your local or national clinical guidelines were enforced by public flogging when not adhered to, would your clinical practice be changed if you were not 'allowed' to use lumbar traction, ultrasound, interferential therapy, laser treatments and TENS?

WHAT DO CLINICAL GUIDELINES SAY ABOUT THE MOST COMMONLY USED PHYSIOTHERAPY TREATMENTS FOR LBP?

In three words – 'not very much'!

At present there still exists a gap in the literature with regard to investigating the opinions of UK physiotherapy clinicians in relation to clinical guidelines and the management of LBP.

Although many clinical guidelines exist in relation to the management of LBP (see Table 2.1) there are significant gaps in the literature when the role of physiotherapy in this management is investigated with minimal physiotherapy input evident in these guidelines (CSP 2004b, Shekelle at al 1999, Woolf 1999).

The systematic reviews in regard to general treatment recommendations for LBP (Table 9.2) can be used to support the research evidence in support of the clinical guidelines related to LBP (Assendelft et al 2003, Furlan et al 2004, Gibson & Waddell 2006, Hagen et al 2004, Karjalainen et al 2003, Khadilkar et al) (Table 9.1).

WHAT CLINICAL GUIDELINES HAVE BEEN PRODUCED IN RELATION TO THE MANAGEMENT OF LBP?

Clinical guidelines for the management and treatment of LBP are plentiful (see Table 9.2).

The clinical guidelines referred to in Table 9.2 have been produced to *aid clinicians* in the management of LBP, offering guidance as to what is seen by experts in the field as the most clinically effective means of managing LBP.

Clinical guidelines for LBP report on common themes from a sound evidence base.

Recurring recommendations from these guidelines include encouraging patients:

- To avoid bed rest
- To receive active treatments
- To avoid passive therapies where possible
- To receive necessary primary care sooner rather than later
- The recognition of red flags as a means of raising suspicion of serious spinal pathology

(Airaksinen et al 2004, Bekkering et al 2003, Bogduk 2000, Burton et al 2004, DHTA 2000, Grimmer et al 2003, Hutchinson et al 1999, Koes et al 2001, van Tulder et al 2004b).

The assessment and treatment of yellow flags: which, as we know from Chapter 4, are psychosocial factors that can increase the risk of a patient with acute LBP developing prolonged pain and disability and affecting work and social circumstances, (Accident Compensation Corporation 2003) are less frequently cited in these guidelines. See the in-depth section in the New Zealand guidelines as the gold standard example of yellow flags and the management of LBP.

www.nzgg.org.nz/guidelines/0072/tcc1038_col.pdf

HISTORICAL PERSPECTIVE OF LBP GUIDELINES RELATED TO THE MANAGEMENT OF LBP IN THE UK

The Royal Collage of General Practitioners, Prodigy Guidelines and The European Guidelines have recently been the most commonly referred to guidelines in the UK.

Table 9.2 Clinical guidelines for LBP

NAME	COUNTRY	PATIENT GROUP	TARGET AUDIENCE	MAIN RECOMMENDATIONS
Agency for Health Care Policy and Research (AHCPR)	United States (AHCPR 1994)	Acute <12 weeks from onset	Primary care	Low impact aerobics. Manipulation <1/12
National Advisory Committee on Health and Disability	New Zealand (ACC 1997, 2003)	<12 weeks from onset	Primary care	No specific exercise. Manipulation <6/52 useful
Royal College of General Practitioners (RCGP)	United Kingdom (Hutchinson et al 1999)	<12 weeks from onset	Primary care GPs	Exercise useful >6/52 manipulation useful to help non responders
National Health and Medical Research Council	Australia (Bogduk et al 2000)	<12 weeks from onset	Primary care GPs	General exercise useful
Danish Institute for Health Technology Assessment	Denmark (DHTA 2000)	Acute < 12, chronic > 12 weeks	Primary care	Manipulation <1/52. McKenzie diagnosis and treatment

Table 9.2 Cont'd

NAME	COUNTRY	PATIENT GROUP	TARGET AUDIENCE	MAIN RECOMMENDATIONS
Dutch College of General Practice	Netherlands (Bekkering et al 2003)	Acute and chronic	GPs	Exercise >6/52, manipulation <6/52 no use
European Guidelines for LBP	European Commission (2004). For the purpose of this table the European Guidelines are a combination of Airaksinen et al (2004); Burton et al (2004) van Tulder et al (2004b), which made up these guidelines	Acute <12 weeks, chronic >12 weeks	Anybody developing or updating guidelines for LBP, including professional bodies	A biopsychosocial approach by musculoskeletal physiotherapists or osteopaths, or chiropractors. Exercise therapy and manipulation for a short course. Traction, electrotherapy, ultrasound, interferential therapy, laser treatments and TENS are specifically listed as not recommended
PRODIGY Guidance - Back pain – lower	England (NHS, 2005)	Acute <12 weeks, chronic >12 weeks.	Health care professionals	This guidance takes account of the 2004 European Guidelines listed above

Within the UK at present the management of LBP is supported and directed by The European Guidelines and The Prodigy Guidelines. In Scotland the Royal Collage of General Practitioners (RCGP) are still the main clinical guideline in use. This isn't because we are slower at adapting to new things here, but because there has been not that much change in guidelines since the RCGP ones were produced in 1996 and 1999.

The change in practice in the UK for LBP management can be traced back to the early 1990s when the Clinical Standards Advisory Group (CSAG) produced their report on back pain. This was not a clinical guideline as such but more a report that was challenged to consider and advise on UK health services for back pain. Its conclusion was that NHS services for back pain at that time were designed mainly for the minority of patients with serious spinal disease, who required specialist investigation or treatment or consideration of surgery. As we know this was a lot of emphasis on quite a small number of patients. Just look at some of the main recommendations from the CSAG report. This report is over 13 years old, but have any of the newer, shinier clinical guidelines added a huge amount of information to help us manage LBP? It is recommended that you revisit the CSAG recommendations again and then compare them to the other guidelines listed below.

OVERVIEW OF CSAG MANAGEMENT GUIDELINES FOR ACUTE BACK PAIN

The CSAG conclusions were that more specialist services should continue to focus on those more potentially serious presentations and that new services should be designed to manage the vast majority of LBP who did not require surgery, imaging etc.

Clinical guidelines were developed jointly with the US guidelines in an appendix to the CSAG Report. However the thorny issue of ownership of these guidelines led to the production of the multidisciplinary Royal College of General Practitioners (RCGP) guidelines. The professional bodies of GPs, orthopaedic surgeons, chiropractors and osteopaths were all represented

Box 9.1	**INITIAL CONSULT**
Diagnostic triage	Simple back pain
	Nerve root pain
	Serious spinal pathology
Early management	Simple analgesia
	If symptoms persist for more than a few days arrange physiotherapy
	Encourage active exercise/physical activity
	Discourage bed rest
	Encourage early activity as not being harmful. Reduces pain and benefits function
	Psychosocial; management is crucial
	Promote early return to work

Biopsychosocial assessment at 6 weeks if not improving

Active rehabilitation programme

Secondary referral for further input if symptoms continue to persist

Final outcome measure: maintain productive activity; reduce work loss
(CSAG 1992)

and endorsed them. It is still open to discussion just how much grassroots involvement was courted in the development of these guidelines. Although these guidelines were distributed throughout the UK, separate funding of the Scottish and Northern Irish health services did produce some distribution difficulties. (So if you have difficultly disseminating your local guidelines do not take it personally!)

RCGP LBP GUIDELINES

Within the United Kingdom, The Royal Collage of General Practitioners (RCGP) Clinical Guidelines for the Management of Acute Low Back Pain (Hutchison et al 1999) are perhaps the most well known guidelines underpinning the overall management and clinical practice of LBP. The RCGP guidelines have consequently become the foundations of LBP management within the NHS (Pinnington et al 2004, Waddell 1998).

The RCGP guidelines were planned to provide evidence-based recommendation for the management of LBP, in the UK, in a multidisciplinary framework that was exposed to reviews and local implementation.

It strongly advocated the use of a 'diagnostic triage' in the assessment of acute LBP (see Fig. 9.1). Patients are categorized as having 'simple LBP', 'nerve root pain', or 'serious spinal pathology' (Waddell 2004).

Quick access to treatment for patients with a 2-week history of LBP who were experiencing their first onset of LBP was encouraged.

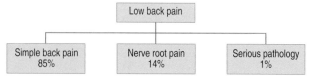

FIG 9.1 Diagnostic triage of LBP.

PRODIGY GUIDELINES

The PRODIGY Guidelines for LBP (NHS 2005) have superseded the RCGP guidelines in England. These guidelines take account of the 2004 European Guidelines for the management of (i) acute simple low back pain in primary care, (ii) chronic simple low back pain, (iii) the prevention of low back pain, and (iv) the diagnosis and treatment of pelvic girdle pain (Airaksinen et al 2004, Burton et al 2004, van Tulder et al 2004b, Vleeming et al 2004).

Full access can easily be found at www.cks.library.nhs.uk/back_pain_lower.

The PRODIGY guidelines cover the symptomatic management of simple low back pain. It includes acute, sub-acute, and chronic low back pain in children, adolescents and adults, and it includes low back pain with and without pain due to nerve root compression. These guidelines are best reviewed in conjunction with the EUROPEAN GUIDELINES discussed below.

EUROPEAN GUIDELINES

Summary of recommendations for acute non-specific LBP

1. Diagnosis

Full history and examination should be carried out.

Identify possible serious spinal pathology or nerve root symptoms, carrying out more extensive neurological examination if deemed necessary.

Undertake diagnostic triage at the first assessment as basis for management decisions.

Be aware of psychosocial factors from an early stage.

Diagnostic imaging tests (including X-rays and MRI) are not routinely indicated for non-specific low back pain.

2. Treatments

Give adequate information and reassure the patient.

Bed rest should be discouraged.

Advise patients to stay active and continue normal daily activities including work if possible.

Check that the patient has been prescribed medication for pain relief; first choice paracetamol, second choice NSAIDs. Important this is taken at regular intervals.

Consider (referral for) spinal manipulation for patients who are failing to return to normal activities.

Multidisciplinary treatment programmes in occupational settings may be an option for workers with sub-acute low back pain and sick leave for more than 4–8 weeks.

van Tulder M, Becker A, Bekkering T et al 2004b European guidelines for the management of acute non-specific low back pain in primary care. European Commission, Research Directorate General. www.backpaineurope.org

Summary of the concepts of diagnosis in chronic low back pain (CLBP)

1. Physical examination and case history

The use of diagnostic triage.

The assessment of yellow flags.

Spinal palpation tests, soft tissue tests and segmental range of motion or straight leg raising tests in the diagnosis of non-specific CLBP cannot be recommended

2. Conservative treatments

Cognitive behavioural therapy, supervised exercise therapy, brief educational.

Interventions for non-specific CLBP can be considered.

Back schools (for short-term improvement), and short courses of manipulation/mobilization can also be considered. The use of physical therapies (heat/cold, traction, laser, ultrasound, short wave, interferential, massage, corsets) *cannot be recommended*.

TENS *is not recommended*.

3. Pharmacological treatments

The short-term use of NSAIDs and weak opioids can be recommended for pain relief.

4. Invasive treatments

Acupuncture cannot be recommended for non-specific CLBP.

Airaksinen O, Brox J I, Cedraschi C et al 2004 European guidelines for the management of chronic non-specific low back pain.

European Commission, Research Directorate General.http://www.backpaineurope.org

Summary of the concepts of prevention in low back pain (LBP)

> The general nature and course of commonly experienced LBP means that there is limited scope for preventing its incidence (first-time onset).
>
> Prevention should be focused on the reduction of the impact and consequences of LBP.
>
> There is considerable scope for the prevention of the consequences of LBP – e.g. episodes (recurrence), care seeking, disability, and work loss.
>
> There is limited valid evidence for numerous aspects of prevention in LBP.
>
> Prevention in LBP will probably require a cultural shift in the way LBP is managed including societal as well as individual concerns.
>
> The most promising approaches seem to involve physical activity/exercise and appropriate (biopsychosocial) education.

Burton A K, Balagué F, Cardon G et al 2004 European guidelines for prevention in low back pain. European Commission, Research Directorate General. www.backpaineurope.org

The PRODIGY Guidelines (NHS 2005), should really be read in conjunction with the wide ranging European Guidelines for acute, chronic and recurrent LBP (Airaksinen et al 2004, Burton et al 2004, van Tulder et al 2004b). Both of these guidelines make it explicitly clear that some physiotherapy modalities, such as:

- Lumbar traction
- Ultrasound
- Interferential therapy
- Laser treatments
- TENS

should not be recommended due to the lack of research evidence as to their clinical effectiveness.

CASE STUDY 9.1

A 45-year-old patient with a 7-month history of central LBP is in the department. Examination reveals loss of lumbar extension. There is no neurological deficit. There are other red flags. She was referred by her GP for acupuncture and the lady is insistent that she receives some acupuncture for her pain. She was given a course of acupuncture 6 years ago in your department and after 10 sessions of acupuncture and a graded exercise programme her symptoms cleared up. She can't remember the exercises from before and is very cautious about moving her spine.

   You know from clinical guidelines that acupuncture for simple mechanical chronic LBP has no evidence even though it 'worked' on that patient previously.

QUESTIONS ON CASE STUDY 9.1

Q1.

How do you decide which treatment to offer or not offer her?

Q2.

How would you justify your decision to yourself, your practice educator (if you are a student), the patient and the GP?

Q3.

Do you take the 'it worked in the past approach' for an easy life?

Q4.

What other factors could have helped symptoms clear up 6 years ago?

Q5.

What potential problems could arise if you choose the 'wrong' approach?

THE POTENTIAL CONFLICT BETWEEN CLINICAL GUIDELINES AND 'TRADITIONAL PHYSIOTHERAPY' FOR LBP

In many of the 1000 RCTs carried out recently the benefits of this 'traditional physiotherapy' were evaluated or compared against other interventions for LBP. Often this 'traditional physiotherapy' was seen as less effective than the 'other modalities' (Burton et al 1999, Frost et al 2004, Hay et al 2005, van Tulder et al 2004a). Potential conflict can arise in the public's eye when this is picked up by the media.

‼ CLINICAL CHALLENGE 9.6

Published literature, either from physiotherapy studies or other medical studies, regularly refers to 'traditional physiotherapy'.

From your own anecdotal evidence, what of sort of physiotherapy treatment do you see generally offered to patients with LBP?

Does it sit in line with the evidence base or more with the 'traditional physiotherapy'?

A prime example of this is the furore from the widely publicised randomized control trial by Helen Frost et al (2004). This paper compared 'traditional' physiotherapy (based from Foster et al 1999) to thorough assessment and advice on self-management. The results showed traditional physiotherapy to be *no more effective* than the advice and self-management. This led to the following newspaper headlines:

'Physiotherapy for back pain is a waste of time and a poor use of NHS money.' (Bosley 2004 in The Guardian)

'Physiotherapy for LBP no better than advice' (Daily Mail 2004)

> ## ‼ CLINICAL CHALLENGE 9.7
>
> These newspaper headlines were in relation to Helen Frost's article in 2004, which caused much interest!
>
> In your opinion, are the headline writers accurate in their description of physiotherapy?
>
> If yes…how?
>
> If no…then why?
>
> Check out Helen's article to see whether her article was so contentious by possibly being very close to the truth.
>
> Frost H, Lamb S, Doll H, Carver P, Stewart-Brown S 2004 Randomized controlled trial of physiotherapy compared with advice for low back pain. British Medical Journal 329:708-714.

Can you imagine the potential issues that this might have in the following scenarios?

• An already anxious patient has just sat in the waiting area reading the Mail or Guardian report. How well do you think your impending treatment session will go now?

• Your local NHS manager has just listened to the radio discussion of this then turned their attention to a recently submitted business plan for extra physiotherapy staffing?

(There really was a discussion on Radio 2 at lunchtime the day the report was released. Not helped by a physiotherapist phoning in to show Jeremy Vine just how good physiotherapy was for LBP by offering him acupuncture and massage!)

This opinion that physiotherapy is *not cost effective or not of much use* is in conflict with recent government legislation or professional demands. These non-medical opinions are inaccurate and are based on poor interpretation of possibly outdated research based on 'traditional physiotherapy'.

This sort of representation in the public eye can only serve to lower the public opinion of physiotherapy management of LBP. This will have a knock-on effect to the successful management of patients with LBP.

How will an already anxious patient respond if they knew about these headlines just before they came to you for assessment? (See yellow flags chapter.)

SUMMARY OF CLINICAL GUIDELINES

In the UK we have been bombarded with guidelines to manage LBP since the birth of the CSAG report. How much these newer guidelines have added to the care of LBP is open to debate. We are guided wisely by these clinical guidelines, which have been developed by extremely educated people with patients' interest at heart. These guidelines have without doubt brought about a sea change in how we all manage LBP, certainly to the benefit of patients and have added to our clinical expertise. Thousands of studies have tried to evaluate the effectiveness of LBP treatments too, but to no clear consensus on what is the most effective treatment. We are now well on the road to proclaiming that we practice evidence-based medicine when managing LBP….or are we?

Mmmm. Maybe not quite in the fast lane just as much as we thought, while there is still one glaring omission that needs to be addressed.

Just how much have individual patient's values and expectations been considered in the development of these guidelines, which now so much shape our day to day management of LBP?

I would venture to suggest very, very little. So how can we say that our management of LBP is truly evidence based if we have excluded patients' values and beliefs? As the literature has previously shown this lack of consultation and involvement among medical professionals can lead to disillusionment and resistance to changing clinical practice (CSP 2004b, Grimmer et al 2003, Moore & Jull 2003, Shekelle at al 1999, van Tulder et al 2001, Woolf et al 1999). What about patients?

EVIDENCE-BASED MEDICINE

WHAT IS EVIDENCE-BASED MEDICINE?

I am sure I have used this term before! Used a lot by NHS managers and budget holders. Evidence-based medicine (EBM) is 'the conscientious, explicit and judicious use of current best evidence in making decisions about the care of individual patients' (Sackett et al 1996).

Put simply, it is the continuous integration of:
- BEST RESEARCH EVIDENCE
- CLINICAL EXPERTISE
- PATIENT'S UNIQUE SET OF VALUES AND EXPECTATIONS (See Fig. 9.2)

Evidence-based medicine is not a recipe book to practice medicine.

(What, no secret cure from the Differential Diagnosis chapter and now this. What sort of self help book is this??!!)

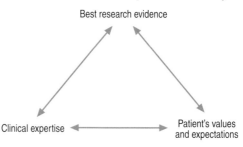

FIG 9.2 Evidence-based medicine.

EBM is a process that enables you to integrate the three aspects above. We have all been told in studies or from reading reviews *that unless your treatment has masses of sound clinical evidence behind it then it is not worth doing.*

This is not just what practising EBM is all about. Does this shock you?

Undoubtedly the more valid and reliable external scientific evidence you have about a certain physiotherapy treatment for LBP, the better. This evidence, nevertheless, cannot fully replace your own clinical expertise. You will still require to weigh up various factors before deciding whether this evidence matches your patient's clinical presentation and preferences, and thus whether your chosen treatment should be applied.

Take the example shown in Figures 9.3, 9.4 and 9.5.

Your patient has LBP and referred pain into their calf and during the subjective and objective assessments has shown a directional preference towards extension (their leg pain centralizes during repeated extension movements). There is no obvious neurological deficit and no red flags of any clinical significance. The only cloud on your sunny prognostic horizon is the fact the patient attended 2 years back for ten sessions of ultrasound (U/S) given to them while lying prone. Their symptoms cleared up over the 3 months they were attending.

You are working with a senior member of staff who is proficient in the McKenzie Diagnosis and Therapy (MDT) approach to managing LBP. After discussing the case with them you plan a treatment based upon extension in lying exercises (EIL) 12 repetitions every 2 hours.

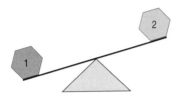

FIG 9.3 Best research evidence.

Figure 9.3 shows that Box 1 (MDT) has a significant heavier body of best research evidence than Box 2 (U/S). However, you are still a fresh-eyed clinician with only limited exposure to MDT and actually probably spend a good few hours on U/S at university and have a significant knowledge of the workings of the flashing machine, so you are not too sure (Fig. 9.4).

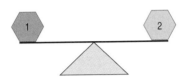

FIG 9.4 Clinical expertise.

Your patient on the other hand has only good things to say about U/S and the thought of carrying out exercises on such a regular basis fills them with horror. To the patient (Fig. 9.5) the weight of evidence based on their unique set of values and circumstance is for the passive heat treatment.

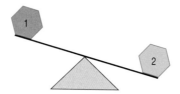

FIG 9.5 The patient's values and expectations.

You are presented now with a unique set of circumstances for this patient. You may spend some time checking Ovid databases for evidence to show patients who present with the centralization/peripheralization phenomena tend to respond well to specific exercises, however your clinical expertise to date is leaving you undecided, which is not being helped by your patient's expectations.

Like some massive game of jenga you are left with a precarious balancing act (Fig. 9.6).

One wrong move and:

(a) The patient will lose all confidence in you, fail to attend, get better anyhow then reappear a few months later with a recurrence of their leg pain.

(b) You will lose confidence in your developing diagnostic skills.

(Just think how much knowledge you have required and how much skill as a clinician you need to have already had to rule out red flags, reach some sort of diagnostic triage, identified yellow flags, asked intimate questions about bladder and bowel function, carried out a thorough neurological assessment, reassured, placated, explained, completed an excellent subjective and objective assessment to reach a loose differential diagnosis of a disc derangement that will be abolished swiftly with a simple extension-based regimen!)

HOW DO I PRACTICE EBM THEN?

Like many buzz words or hot topics in the NHS, EBM is used widely, dangerously and often without due consideration for

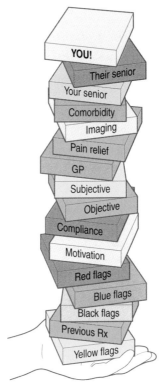

FIG 9.6 The difficult balancing act that is the management of LBP.

what it actually means. The pocket book by Straus et al (see below) is as good a place as any to start from.

- But also think of the three main components of EBM: best research evidence, clinical expertise and patient's unique set of values and expectations.

Best research evidence

Look at journals on the web. Use OVID databases. Never just rely on your own professional journal. Pick a few key journals in each speciality and set up alerts. In LBP a starting point would be:

- *Spine*
- *The Spine Journal*
- *Manual Therapy*
- *Pain*
- *Physical Therapy*
- *Australian Journal of Physiotherapy*
- *European Spine Journal*

Don't just agree with everything written too. Most of you reading this book will be recent graduates. Remember the hours you spent critically appraising articles for projects and final thesis? Well you are allowed to use these skills when qualified or in a clinical setting too!

Journal Clubs that achieve something tangible are an excellent way to discuss this evidence and impress/intimidate seniors. Pick a topic area and review a handful of articles in the subject. Write up the results, disseminate information too! *Back Chat* is the newsletter of the GGBPS and is always keen and willing to print interesting literature reviews (www.nhsggc.org.uk/ggbps). There will be others too. The very worst thing you can do is keep it secret. Doesn't matter if it is not a Cochrane review, but it is applicable to your area, type of patient and staff make up and worth sharing, especially between colleagues in your own Health Board, Primary Care Trust or even sitting next to you!

Is this best evidence applicable to your area of work? Yellow flags are an integral part of the assessment of LBP. Does where you work have access to clinical psychology to manage them, is there training for yellow flags? Never assume those more senior than you have flagged this up. Audit it, review it, write it up and send it to somebody who can do something about it. And keep doing it until something is done or you are in a more senior position to do so. Most of these areas have a sufficiently strong evidence base to push this through….if where you work really practises the EBM model they preach!

If you work in the UK then all this work can also be useful for your HPC registration when chosen.

Clinical expertise

ALL GRADES of physiotherapist should be able to contribute to the local EBM practised around LBP. The best areas where this happens are those where staff share the personal strengths whether it is an undergrad with a recent course work or a more senior staff member just finished their MSC. Remember you have many years to work and remain relatively sane and enthused; so if that isn't what happens where you work just now………

Of course your clinical expertise will change as the years go on. Most undergraduate training prepares you for reflecting on your practice and appraising your decision making. There is no shame in admitting you haven't a clue with certain patients. Revisit this book regularly and review your answers to the various clinical challenges. Bet you there is a vast difference, and improvement every time you complete an outpatient placement or rotation.

Choose your postgrad training courses wisely. There are enough articles and text references in this book to start this process.

Patient's unique set of values and expectations

This is the easy part!

If you have read this book then by now you will know all about a thorough assessment, addressing yellow flags, contextualizing questions, involving patients in the decision process, asking them what the want, how to achieve it, been honest about causes (or lack of them) of pain, how it goes away, how best to achieve this etc! This means you have immediately addressed each patient's unique set of values and expectations. Bet you are the first medical professional to spend so much time with these unique set of circumstances.

Next challenge. How to add to the changing face of LBP management. See the next chapter for some pointers.

TAKE HOME MESSAGE

At least make sure your chosen treatment is having some sort of justifiable physiological response to the symptoms you see before you!

Clinical studies exist to present evidence on the study group used. Again, they are not the only way.

Clinical guidelines exist to help practitioners and patients decide on the most appropriate and effective healthcare for specific clinical conditions. They are not the only way.

Clinical guidelines can help you to deal with dilemmas over what treatment to give the patient and what treatment they want. Again, an honest approach by at least offering and discussing guidelines with patients is a good starting point.

There is no cure to LBP, and more guidelines do not necessarily mean they have anything new to say.

EBM is not just about having valid and reliable evidence for your chosen treatment, but includes your expertise and patient's values and expectations – DON'T FORGET!

It is your responsibility as an autonomous physiotherapy practitioner to challenge clinical guidelines and published research, as well as agree and use them for support. It is also your responsibility to add to these areas in the future.

RECOMMENDED ADDITIONAL READING/REFERENCES

The Back Book (2nd edn. The Stationery Office, Norwich www.tso. co.uk)

Airaksinen O, Brox J I, Cedraschi C et al 2004 European guidelines for the management of chronic non-specific low back pain. European Commission, Research Directorate General. http://www. backpaineurope.org

Burton A K, Balagué F, Cardon G et al 2004 European guidelines for prevention in low back pain. European Commission, Research Directorate General. www.backpaineurope.org

Evidence Based Medicine Guidelines accessible via http://ebmg.wiley.com/ebmg/ltk.koti (you will require an ATHENS password for full access)

Hutchinson A, Waddell G, Feder G 1999 Clinical guidelines for the management of acute low back pain. London: Royal College of General Practitioners; www.rcgp.org.uk

NHS 2005 Prodigy Guidance – back pain – lower. www.prodigy.nhs.uk/guidance.asp?gt=Backpain-lower

Straus S E, Richardson W S et al 2005 Evidence Based Medicine: How To Teach and Practice EBM, 3rd edn. Elsevier, Edinburgh.

van Tulder M, Becker A, Bekkering T et al 2004 European guidelines for the management of acute non-specific low back pain in primary care. European Commission, Research Directorate General. www.backpaineurope.org

REFERENCES

Accident Compensation Corporation (ACC) 1997, 2003 New Zealand acute low back pain guide, incorporating the guide to assessing psychological yellow flags in acute low back pain. www.nzgg.og.nz/guidelines/0072/albp_guide_col.pdf (accessed 25/05/07).

Agency for Health Care Policy and Research 1994 Acute Low Back Problems in Adults. Clinical Practice Guideline Number 14 Public Health Service, US Department of Health and Human Services Rockville, Maryland.

Airaksinen O, Brox J I, Cedraschi C et al 2004 European guidelines for the management of chronic non-specific low back pain. European Commission, Research Directorate General.http://www.backpaineurope.org (last accessed 29/08/07).

Assendelft W J J, Morton S C, Yu E I et al 2003 Spinal manipulative therapy for low-back pain. The Cochrane Database of Systematic Reviews. The Cochrane Collaboration. John Wiley.

Assendelft W J J, Morton S C, Yu E I et al 2003 Spinal manipulative therapy for low back pain. Annals of Internal Medicine 138(11):871-881.

Barnett A G, Underwood M R, Vickers M R 1999 Effect of UK national guidelines on services to treat patients with acute low back pain: follow up questionnaire survey. BMJ 318:919-920.

Battie M C, Cherkin D C, Dunn R 1994 Managing low back pain: attitudes and treatment preferences of physical therapists. Physical Therapy. 74:219-226.

BEAM 2004 UK back pain exercise and manipulation (UK BEAM) Trial Team randomized trial: cost effectiveness of physical treatments for back pain in primary care. British Medical Journal 329(7479):1381-1387.

Bekkering G E, Hendriks H J M, Koes B W 2003 Dutch Physiotherapy Guidelines for Low Back Pain Physiotherapy 89(2):82-96.

Bogduk N Draft evidence based clinical guidelines for the management of acute low back pain. National Health and Medical Research Council, Australia, 2000 (URL: http://www.health.gov.au/: 80/nhmrc/media/2000rel/pain.htm) (last accessed 29/05/07).

Borkan J M, Cherkin D C 1996 An agenda for primary care research on low back pain. Spine 21:2880-2884.

Bosley S 2004 Physiotherapy doesn't work for back pain. Guardian newspaper 24th September www.theguardian.co.uk (last accessed 21/05/2007).

Burton A K, Waddell G, Tillotson K M et al1999 Information and advice to patients with back pain can have a positive effect: a randomized controlled trial of a novel educational booklet in primary care Spine 24:2484-2491.

Burton A K, Balagué F, Cardon G et al 2004 European guidelines for prevention in low back pain. European Commission, Research Directorate General. www.backpaineurope.org (last accessed 29/04/07).

Chartered Society of Physiotherapy 2004 Making Physiotherapy Count. A Range of Quality Assured Services. Chartered Society of Physiotherapy, London.

Chou R 2005 Evidence-based medicine and the challenge of low back pain: where are we now? Pain Practice 5(3):153-178.

Daily Mail 2004 Frequent physiotherapy is no better than advice www.dailymail.co.uk 24th September 2004 (last accessed 21/05/07).

Danish Health Technology Assessment (DHTA) 1999 Low Back Pain – frequency, management and prevention from an HTA perspective. Danish Health Technology Assessment 1999;1(1). http://www.sst.dk/Applikationer/cemtv/publikationer/ docs/Low-back%20pain/LowBackPain.pdf (last accessed 29/08/05)

Daykin A R, Richardson B 2004 Physiotherapists' pain beliefs and their influence on the management of patients with chronic low back pain. Spine 29(7):783-795.

Dey P D, Simpson C W R, Collins SI et al 2004 Implementation of RCGP guidelines for acute low back pain: a cluster randomized controlled trial. British Journal of General Practice 54:33-37.

Deyo R A, Phillips W R 1996 Low back pain: a primary care challenge. Spine 21:2826-2832.

Engel G L 1977 The need for a new medical model: a challenge for biomedicine. Science 196(4286):129-136.

European Commission 2004 Low Back Pain. Guidelines for its Management www.backpaineurope.org

Ferguson F C, Webster V, Brownlee M 2008 A Delphi study investigating consensus among expert physiotherapists in relation to the management of low back pain. Musculosketal Care (in press).

Field M J, Lohr K N (eds) 1992 Institute of Medicine Committee to Advise the Public Health Service on Clinical Practice Guidelines. Clinical Practice Guidelines: directions for a new work programme. Washington (DC): National Academy Press.

Foster N, Thompson K, Baxter J M 1999 Management of non-specific low back pain by therapists in Britain and Ireland. Spine 24(13):1332-1342.

Frost H, Lamb S, Doll H et al 2004 Randomized controlled trial of physiotherapy compared with advice for low back pain. BMJ 329:708-714.

Furlan A D, van Tulder M W, Cherkin D C et al 2006 Acupuncture and dry-needling for low back pain. The Cochrane Database of Systematic Reviews. The Cochrane Collaboration. John Wiley.

Gibson J N A, Waddell G 2006 Surgical interventions for lumbar disc prolapse. The Cochrane Database of Systematic Reviews. The Cochrane Collaboration. John Wiley.

Gracey J H, McDonough S M, Baxter G D 2001 Physiotherapy management of low back pain: a survey of current practice in Northern Ireland. Spine 27(4):406-411.

Grimmer K, Milanese S, Bialocerkowski A 2003 Clinical guidelines for low back pain: a physiotherapy perspective. Physiotherapy Canada 55:185-194.

Hagen K B, Hilde G, Jamtvedt G et al 2004 Bed rest for acute low-back pain and sciatica. The Cochrane Database of Systematic Reviews. The Cochrane Collaboration. John Wiley.

Hay E M, Mullis R, Lewis M et al 2005 Comparison of physical treatments versus a brief pain management programme for back pain in primary care: a randomized clinical trial in physiotherapy practice Lancet 365:2024-2030.

Hayden J A, van Tulder MW, Malmivaara A et al 2005 Exercise therapy for treatment of non-specific low back pain. The Cochrane Database of Systematic Reviews. The Cochrane Collaboration. John Wiley.

Hutchinson A, Waddell G, Feder G 1999 Clinical Guidelines for the Management of Acute Low Back Pain. London: Royal College of General Practitioners; www.rcgp.org.uk

Jadad AR, Moher M, Browman GP et al 2000 Systematic reviews and meta-analyses on treatment of asthma: critical evaluation. BMJ 320:537-540.

Karjalainen K, Malmivaara A, van Tulder MW et al 2003 Multidisciplinary biopsychosocial rehabilitation for subacute low-back pain among working age adults. The Cochrane Database of Systematic Reviews. The Cochrane Collaboration. John Wiley.

Khadilkar A, Milne S, Brosseau L et al 2005 Transcutaneous electrical nerve stimulation for the treatment of chronic low back pain: a systematic review. Spine 30(23):2657-2666.

Li L C, Bombardier C 2001 Physical therapy management of low back pain: an exploratory survey of therapist approaches. Physical Therapy 81:1018-1028.

Long A, Donelson R, Fung T 2004 Does it matter which exercise? a randomized control trial of exercise for low back pain. Spine 29(23):2593-2602.

McKenzie R A 2005 The myth of acute low back pain. New Zealand Family Physician 32(2):125-126.

Mikhail C, Korner-Bitensky N, Rossignol M et al 2005 Physical therapists' use of interventions with high evidence of effectiveness in the management of a hypothetical typical patient with acute low back pain. Physical Therapy 85(11):1151-1167.

Moore A, Jull G 2003 Clinical guideline development. Manual Therapy 8(4):193-194.

NHS 2005 Prodigy Guidance – back pain – lower. www.prodigy.nhs.uk/guidance.asp?gt=Backpain-lower (accessed 10/08/06)

Ostelo R W, Stomp-van den Berg S G, Vlaeyen J W 2003 Health care providers' attitudes and beliefs towards chronic low back pain: the development of a questionnaire. Manual Therapy 8:214-222.

Oxman A D, Guyatt G H 1991 Validation of an index of the quality of review articles. Journal of Clinical Epidemiogy 44:1271-1278.

Pengel L H M, Herbert R D, Maher C G et al 2003 Acute low back pain: systematic review of its prognosis. BMJ 327(7410):323-327.

Pinnington M A, Miller J, Stanley I 2004 An evaluation of prompt access to physiotherapy in the management of low back pain in primary care. Family Practice 21(4):372-380.

Sackett D L, Rosenberg W M, Gray J A et al 1996 Evidence based medicine: what it is and what it isn't. BMJ 312(7023):71-72.

Scottish Executive, Department of Health 2003 Partnership for Care. Scotland's Health White Paper http//www.scotland.gov.uk/library3/health/ronh.pdf. (accessed 18/03/2005).

Scottish Executive, Department of Health 2005 Delivering for Health. www.scotland.gov.uk/Topics/Health/care/communitynursing/deliveringforhealth

Scottish Office, Department of Health 1998 Designed to Care: renewing the National Health Service in Scotland. http//www.scotland.gov.uk (last accessed 01/11/06).

Shekelle P G, Woolf S H, Eccles M 1999 Developing guidelines. BMJ 318:59-596.

Turk D C, Flor H 1984 Etiological theories and treatments for chronic back pain. II. Psychological models and interventions. Pain 19:209-233.

van Tulder M W, Koes B W, Bouter L M 1997 Low back pain in primary care. Effectiveness of diagnostic and therapeutic interventions. Amsterdam: Faculteit der Geneeskunde VU. EMGO-Instituut. Cited Scher et al 2000.

van Tulder M W, Anitti M D, Esmail R et al 2000 Exercise therapy for low back pain: a systematic review within the Cochrane collaboration back review group. Spine 2(21):2784-2796.

van Tulder M W, Malmivaara A, Email R et al 2004a Exercise therapy for low back pain (review). The Cochrane Database of Systematic Reviews vol 2.

van Tulder M, Becker A, Bekkering T et al 2004b European guidelines for the management of acute non-specific low back pain in primary care. European Commission, Research Directorate General. www.backpaineurope.org (last accessed 29/08/05).

Vleeming A, Albert H B, Östgaard H et al 2004 European Guidelines for the Diagnosis and Treatment of Pelvic Girdle Pain. www.backpaineurope.org/web/html/wg4_results.html

Waddell G (1998, 2004) The Back Pain Revolution. Churchill Livingstone, Edinburgh

Woolf S H, Grol R, Hutchison A et al 1999 Potential benefits, limitations and harms of clinical guidelines BMJ 318:527-530.

Examples of how specialist services can change the management of LBP

CHAPTER

10

CONTENTS

WORKING BACKS SCOTLAND **200**

AUSTRALIAN STUDY **200**

THE GREATER GLASGOW BACK PAIN SERVICE **201**

AIMS AND OBJECTIVES

Aim: To show the reader how developing new specialist services can positively tackle the problem of LBP

Objectives: By the end of this chapter the reader will:

1. Be aware of some specialist services developed to manage LBP
2. Be able to discuss the background to a back pain service
3. Be aware of how patients enter the Greater Glasgow Back Pain Service
4. Have knowledge of exit routes available to patients with LBP

Remember, all these services and innovations started because one person had an idea, whether it is a politician, orthopaedic surgeon, researcher or in many cases a physiotherapist. These services and innovations are not the end of the line. Like most innovations they are often taken for granted with people nit-picking about this and that, and never fully appreciated until they have stopped. The innovators from all the services discussed would openly admit if you asked that they are not perfect and the best way in which they will have lasting impact is if the next generation of innovators help out, ask awkward questions and challenge the previously unchallenged. Why not you?

WORKING BACKS SCOTLAND

In the mid-1990s, in an attempt to cascade the huge amount of new scientific evidence under-pinning the management of non-specific low back pain, that showed a move from the more traditional model of care promoting rest until the pain got better to a more positive strategy of encouraging and supporting patients to continue ordinary activities as normally as possible and to stay at work or return to work as soon as possible, Working Backs Scotland was launched.

This involved 20 organizations from physiotherapists, GPs and pharmacists.

The campaign's basic message was simple:

• 'Don't take back pain lying down!'

Over 35 000 information packs were distributed, and a radio campaign broadcast nearly 2000 adverts. Population studies suggested 60% penetration and a 20% positive shift in public beliefs.

http://www.workingbacksscotland.scot.nhs.uk/AboutUs/wbs.htm

AUSTRALIAN STUDY

A similar campaign was carried out in two Australian States to bring about a positive impact on population beliefs about back pain and fear-avoidance beliefs. A massive multimedia campaign advised patients with back pain to stay active and exercise, not to rest for prolonged periods, and to remain at work was measured in telephone surveys, and the effect of the campaign on the potential management of low back pain by GPS was assessed by eliciting their likely approach to two hypothetical scenarios in mailed surveys.

This study showed positive beliefs as a result of the campaign from both patients and GPS (Buchbinder et al 2001). Longer term follow up studies have shown maintenance of these beliefs (Buchbinder & Jolly 2007).

THE GREATER GLASGOW BACK PAIN SERVICE: PHYSIOTHERAPY-LED BACK PAIN SERVICE

BACKGROUND

The Greater Glasgow Back Pain Service (GGBPS) is a National Health Service (NHS) funded initiative established in 2002 to provide a service to the population of Glasgow, Scotland (870 000).

- Its initial aim was to set up a dedicated Acute Back Pain Service to implement the RCGP guidelines for the management of patients with acute LBP and to develop the service in response to any changes in professional and legislative demands.

A successful pilot had been carried out in 1999 when 2.5 whole-time equivalent, specialist physiotherapists were employed to establish and run the service, which provided rapid, direct access to physical therapy for the GPs of North East Glasgow in both Primary Care and Acute Trusts.

The GGBPS is led by a Lead Physiotherapist overseeing service organization and the management of all patients with LBP within NHS Greater Glasgow and Clyde (NHSGGC).

Figure 10.1 gives a thorough overview of the GGBPS.

Permanent funding was granted for 10 whole-time equivalent (WTE) Clinical Physiotherapy Specialists, including the Lead Clinician, 2.8 WTE Psychologists to allow appropriate service development and 1.2 WTE administrative and clerical support to provide service support for GGBPS.

- This is a physiotherapy-led and delivered service. It extends beyond the scope of the initial service by integrating the

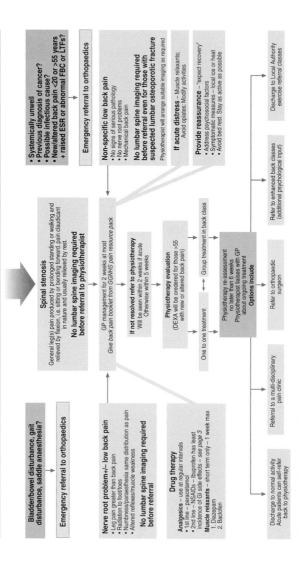

Glasgow Low Back Pain Service

Bladder/bowel disturbance, gait disturbance, saddle anaesthesia?

Emergency referral to orthopaedics

Nerve root problem+/– low back pain
- Leg pain greater than back pain
- Radiation to foot/toes
- Numbness/paraesthesia same distribution as pain
- Altered reflexes/muscle weakness

No lumbar spine imaging required before referral

Drug therapy

Analgesics – use at regular intervals
- 1st line – paracetamol
- 2nd line – NSAIDs – Ibuprofen has least incidence of GI side effects – *see page 3*

Muscle relaxants – short term only – 1 week max
1. Diazepam
2. Baclofen

Spinal stenosis

General leg(s) pain produced by prolonged standing or walking and relieved by flexion, i.e. sitting or bending forward, pain claudicant in nature and usually relieved by rest.

No lumbar spine imaging required before referral to physiotherapist

GP management for 2 weeks at most
Give back pain booklet from GGNHS pain resource pack

If not resolved refer to physiotherapy
Will be seen within 2 weeks if acute
Otherwise within 5 weeks

Physiotherapy evaluation
(DEXA will be ordered for those >55 with new or altered back pain)

One to one treatment ⟷ Group treatment in back class

Physiotherapy re-assessment
no later than 6 weeks
Physiotherapist liaises with GP about ongoing treatment
Options include

- **Systemically unwell**
- **Previous diagnosis of cancer?**
- **Possible infectious cause?**
- **New/altered back pain <20 or >55 years + raised ESR or abnormal FBC or LTFs?**

Emergency referral to orthopaedics

Non-specific low back pain
- No signs of serious pathology
- No nerve root problems
- Mechanical back pain

No lumbar spine imaging required before referral even for those with suspected lumbar osteoporotic fracture
Physiotherapist will arrange suitable imaging as required

If acute distress – Muscle relaxants; Avoid opiates: Modify activities

Provide reassurance – 'expect recovery'
- Address psychosocial factors
- Symptomatic measures – local ice or heat
- Avoid bed rest. Stay as active as possible

Discharge to normal activity
Acute patients can self-refer back to physiotherapy

Referral to a multi-disciplinary pain clinic

Refer to orthopaedic surgeon

Refer to enhanced back classes (additional psychological input)

Discharge to Local Authority exercise referral classes

FIG 10.1 GGBPS overview, 2003.

physiotherapy management of patients with both acute and non-acute LBP.

A key factor of the GGBPS is that it includes all physiotherapists within NHSGGC who manage LBP. This allows a coordinated and consistent approach to the management of LBP in the largest health board in Scotland.

Patients are seen at a number of locations throughout the city and managed in line with the guidance published by Hutchinson et al (1999), which advocates diagnostic triage and rapid access to treatment (< 6 weeks) for acute LBP.

Outcome measures for functional status and pain (Quebec Task Force, Visual Analogue Scale (VAS)) are routinely used. Care pathways for cauda equina, serious red flags, imaging, surgery and psychology referrals have been developed and implemented in conjunction with and approved by local medical specialists and staff fully trained in their use.

EVALUATION

Thorough city-wide statistics in relation to waiting times and number of patients referred to physiotherapy prior to the introduction of the GGBPS are non-existent. It is suggested that this lack of statistics will not be unique to Glasgow.

However, there was enough strong anecdotal evidence from imagers, General Practitioners, Orthopaedic Consultants and physiotherapists plus more locally based statistics to merit the introduction of the pilot study and to provide significant funding to set up the city-wide service.

In the last 4 years an average 7000 patients were seen annually. 85% of acute LBP (n = 3134) are seen within 2 weeks. See Table 10.1 for a breakdown of these figures. In parts of the city the number of plain film lumbar spine X-rays carried out has decreased by 90%.

ENTRY ROUTES

How patients access physiotherapy for their LBP is clearly displayed in Figure 10.2. These entry routes were based on clinical guidelines discussed earlier.

Table 10.1 Breakdown of GGBPS patients, 2005 (with permission of GGBPS)

Overview

56 %	Female			44 %	Male
65 %	Lumbar			35 %	Nerve root
83 %	Insidious onset	10 %	Occupational	7 %	Trauma
65 %	Acute symptoms i.e. <6/52			35 %	Non-acute symptoms >6/12

Accessing GGBPS

36 %	Self refer following GP advice
36 %	GP referral
19 %	Self-referral
5 %	Physiotherapy colleague
4 %	Other

Using Quebec Task Force definitions

4 %	No pain
42 %	Lumbar pain
16 %	Lumbar pain referred to knee
17 %	Lumbar pain referred below the knee
31 %	Lumbar pain referred below the knee with neurological symptoms

Outcome of discharge

63 %	Self care
3 %	Back class
1 %	Orthopaedic surgeon
1 %	GP
1 %	Pain Clinic
21 %	Other (Inc DNA/FTA etc)

Average number of GGBPS contacts

35 %	<2 visits
52 %	<4 visits

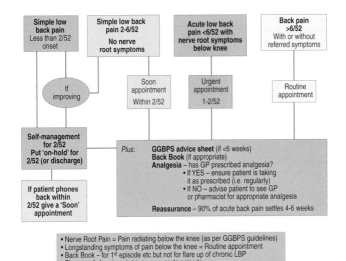

FIG 10.2 Entry routes to GGBPS.

EXIT ROUTES

There are numerous exit routes available for physiotherapists and patients when their course of physiotherapy is complete. These are clearly defined in Figures 10.3 to 10.14.

The average city-wide wait for an X-ray and waiting times for magnetic resonance imaging (MRI) scan and orthopaedic opinions reduced from 40 to around 8 weeks. Financially this reduction in X-rays alone is significant when the average cost of each lumbar spine X-ray is £54.50 (Scottish Health Statistics Information & Statistics Division 2005).

Just 1.2 % (n = 83) were referred for imaging and/or surgical opinion; a similar rate reported by the RCGP for medically led services (Hutchison 1999). Of the number of patients seen exclusively by the specialist team, 80% of patients (n = 2148) reported functional improvement; 90% (n = 2417) reported >= 50% reduction in pain (VAS), 68% (n = 1827) were discharged in <= 3 contacts (1–23 range).

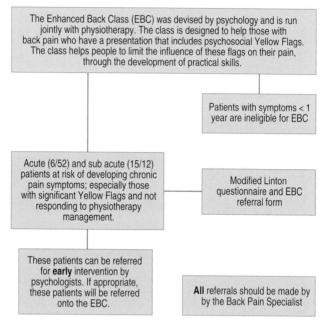

The Enhanced Back Class (EBC) was devised by psychology and is run jointly with physiotherapy. The class is designed to help those with back pain who have a presentation that includes psychosocial Yellow Flags. The class helps people to limit the influence of these flags on their pain, through the development of practical skills.

Patients with symptoms < 1 year are ineligible for EBC

Acute (6/52) and sub acute (15/12) patients at risk of developing chronic pain symptoms; especially those with significant Yellow Flags and not responding to physiotherapy management.

Modified Linton questionnaire and EBC referral form

These patients can be referred for **early** intervention by psychologists. If appropriate, these patients will be referred onto the EBC.

All referrals should be made by by the Back Pain Specialist

FIG 10.3 Psychology (enhanced back class). Figures 10.3 to 10.14 show exit routes from GGBPS, 2006 (with permission of GGBPS).

A patient satisfaction survey of 644 patients carried out in 2005, 2 months after discharge indicated high satisfaction with the service. Audit of service delivery against clinical guidelines showed physiotherapy treatment in line with clinical guidelines and evidence-based practice in 75% of all physiotherapy staff (n = 165).

CONCLUSIONS OF THE EFFECTIVENESS OF GGBPS

Since its introduction, the physiotherapy-led GGBPS has demonstrated significant benefits for patients. They now gain speedier access to equitable, safe and evidence-based care, a service highly valued and, which is achieving proven outcomes.

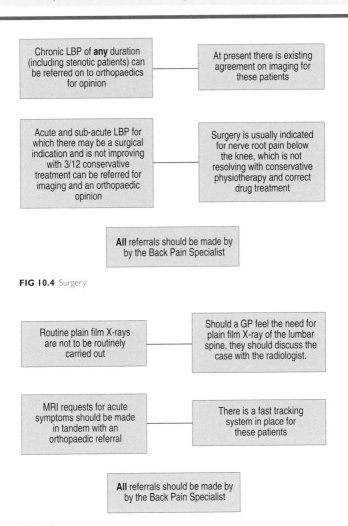

FIG 10.4 Surgery.

FIG 10.5 Imaging.

Working autonomously as primary carers requires physiotherapists to be responsible and accountable for the care they provide. Physiotherapy within the GGBPS has been demonstrated to suggest treatment in line with clinically effective care.

All physiotherapy staff can refer a patient for a DEXA scan if concerned about osteoporosis

Osteoporosis may affect the type of exercise prescribed or if the patients should be referred to an osteoporosis class

FIG 10.6 DEXA.

These exercise classes are designed to help people manage their back pain and return to normal activities. They also aim to prevent recurrence of back problems by helping the person to stay active.

A modified Linton questionnaire should be filled out before referral to these classes; patients scoring > 105 (if working) and > 80 (if not working) should not generally be referred.

FIG 10.7 Physiotherapy-led back class.

Back to basics classes are an easy introduction to exercise and exercise techniques, with non-medical supervision

Suitable for those experiencing back pain or those who want to become more active and combine a range of activities at a lower intensity level

FIG 10.8 Community-led classes.

Patients who are discharged to self care should be told that they can contact their phyiotherapist within two months if the pain returns. After the two months, the patient should access physiotherapy through their local referral clinic.

This standard should be applied to all LBP patients, no matter who is treating them

FIG 10.9 Self care.

Pain Association Scotland (PAS) utllilizes groups which are participant led, and helps to educate them about the causes of pain, the management of and coping with chronic pain.
Patients may attend regulary or only when they need support.
An information leaflet is available for patient information and PAS contact details.

FIG 10.10 Pain Association Scotland (PAS).

The Pain Clinic involves individual assessment and intervention by the appropriate clinician (physiotherapist, psychologist or anaesthetist), or group of clinicians to help the patient cope with their pain

Patients with poor pain management (particularly with chronic pain) may benefit from a multidisciplinary team approach

GGBPS may refer directly to the Pain Clinic
GPs are also able to initiate referral

Some patients with < 6/12 duration of nerve root symptoms may benefit from an early assessment at the Pain Clinic for nerve root blocks or caudal epidurals

All referrals should be made by the Back Pain Specialist

FIG 10.11 Pain clinic.

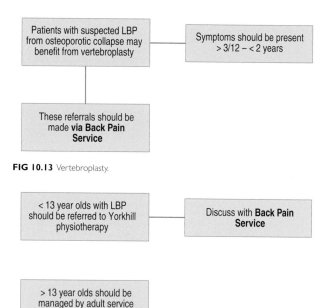

Patients with suspected serious spinal pathology should be referred immediately back to their GP for review, including screening bloods. Serious spinal pathology would include the presence of significant Red Flags such as weight loss and history of cancer.

Cauda Equina Syndrome (CES) is a potential surgical emergency These patients should not be referred back to their GP

They should be managed in line with the GGBPS CES triage chart

FIG 10.12 Back to GP.

Patients with suspected LBP from osteoporotic collapse may benefit from vertebroplasty

Symptoms should be present > 3/12 – < 2 years

These referrals should be made **via Back Pain Service**

FIG 10.13 Vertebroplasty.

< 13 year olds with LBP should be referred to Yorkhill physiotherapy

Discuss with **Back Pain Service**

> 13 year olds should be managed by adult service

FIG 10.14 Paediatric cases.

Comparative studies are required to show if any benefits of the GGBPS can be transferable to other health board areas.

REFERENCES

Buchbinder R, Jolley D 2007 Improvements in general practitioner beliefs and stated management of back pain persist 4.5 years after the cessation of a public health media campaign. Spine 32(5):E156-E162.

Buchbinder R, Jolley D, Wyatt M 2001 Volvo Award Winner in clinical studies: Effects of a media campaign on back pain beliefs and its potential influence on management of low back pain in general practice. Spine 26(23):2535-2542.

Greater Glasgow Back Pain Service 2006 Pathway Document for the Management of Low Back Pain (Unpublished).

Hutchinson A, Waddell G, Feder G 1999 Clinical Guidelines for the Management of Acute Low Back Pain. Royal College of General Practitioners www.rcgp.org.uk

Information Services Division 2006 Scottish Health Service Costs Book Manual www.isdscotland.org

Possible answers to Clinical Challenges and Case Studies

Appendix

The answers on the Clinical Challenges (CC) and Case Studies (CS) are not the only answers. They are only one man's thoughts which give possible solutions to what the answers could be and to provoke and stimulate the reader into expanding the answers and even to challenging them. Not every one has been answered either.

CC 1.1

1. Some benefits could be planning of services, staffing, costs and treatments. Better strategy for the management of LBP. Some pitfalls could be loss of control by clinicians, disagreements over classification.
2. This is very hard indeed. I cannot offer a definitive answer!

CC 1.2

This could involve regular appointments at a GP for a cure and/ or medication. (See Holdsworth & Webster 2007.) Repeated referrals to physiotherapy, orthopaedics, pain clinics. Time off work with financial implications to employer, employee and governments. Ongoing pain management perhaps specialist pain clinics etc.

CC 2.1

The diagnostic triage is a fair representation of my own case-load. However it doesn't necessarily mean it is the best representation of it.

The diagnostic triage is cited in nearly every clinical guideline I have read. Personally I don't know how pleased I would be to be categorized with 85% of people with a similar non-specific problem. Is there a better option? The first few chapters in the superb book by Donelson, *Rapidly Reversible Back Pain*, question this triaging. The categorizing of LBP remains the 'holy grail' of LBP research.

CC 2.2

The obvious red flags present are age (>55 years old) and history of cancer. You could suggest that there is a history of trauma and pain may be constant but until further assessment we wouldn't know if it was constant non-mechanical pain.

I wouldn't be too worried as yet. It is an acute injury. The patient has no right to be better in 2 days. If the injury is relevant you would expect improvement in a few weeks. With all red flags they are monitored and if symptoms do not progress as you would expect then swift referral back to their GP, stating your concerns, is indicated.

There is still an acute inflammatory response ongoing after 2 days.

CC 2.3

Yellow flags. More specifically attitudes, behaviours, beliefs and diagnosis would spring to mind. Just imagine you have been told you have a benign harmless heart problem but there is some sort of abnormal valve that is twisted and out of shape. Which part of that statement from a cardiologist do you remember most of?

Patients are continually told this by some alternative practitioners. Using an X-ray or X-ray vision they are told they have a twisted spine with one leg longer than the other. They generally visit these alternative practitioners when they are in a considerable amount of pain and pay for the pleasure.

CC 2.4

Red flags are applicable to all musculoskeletal conditions (as are yellow flags); with slight variances on red flag questions depending on the area you are applying them to.

CS 3.1

1. Knowing the whole clinical presentation of this particular patient I would say he was handled proficiently and safely by all physiotherapists who saw him.
2. Initially altered urination closely monitored. Second episode trauma, altered bladder function, constant non-mechanical pain.

CS 4.1

Yellow flags should be looked for from the first minute you start to assess a LBP patient. You will find patients all react differently to pain and as such yellow flags can develop at different times. Patients with a recurrent problem can often show yellow flags earlier in the course of a new episode of LBP. This is because in spite of careful self management they feel disappointed that they have had a recurrence.

Lesley has medical training so you may feel that mentioning psychosocial issues could antagonize her. Careful explanation of the whole process can go a long way to avoiding this. Remember not to undersell your role in yellow flag management and have the confidence to be aware that you probably have more knowledge on this area than most other medical professionals. Lesley has also been told by a well meaning GP, without an MRI, that she has a slipped disc. This may then confuse her when you try to reassure her that things normally will clear up in a few weeks with physiotherapy. Lesley's own experience of LBP is in A&E, where patients are normally in severe distress and she has little exposure to patients recovering from LBP without passive (and often justified and effective) medical intervention.

It is quite often difficult to put people at ease about yellow flags. It takes practice and the more you do talk about it the (like most things) better you will get. Gail has only had her symptoms for 1 week so you may not directly even need to broach the subject. Positive reinforcement of attitudes, behaviours, returning to normal activities and work are often integral parts of any physiotherapy assessment.

The longer you are off work with LBP the less likely it is you will ever return. If there really is a physical problem at work you should discuss it with Lesley; every worker has a right to a safe working environment through the Health and Safety at Work Act.

CS 4.2

It is possible that Donald may not be overly pleased. His mood is low to start with and questioning him on some psychosocial component to his problem may be too much! However, you will be surprised just how many patients are relieved that their symptoms are 'not all in my head', when you gently suggest there may be more than physical factors affecting their recovery.

Bob is clearly showing yellow flags around A, B, D, E, F and W. But why guess? The Linton LBP screening tool available in the New Zealand guidelines is a validated tool for gauging yellow flags – see recommended reading section in Chapter 4.

Bob has already told you he is experiencing low mood and problems at home. Often a partner is very worried that their partner is in severe pan and has changed their personality. The first sign of this is that they become anxious which can manifest itself in anger and resentment towards the LBP patients. We are not counsellors but discussing the idea of yellow flags with Bob, who could maybe mention these to his wife, is a start. It is tricky though and he could easily kick off at you. I have treated many Bob's and cautiously and carefully is the way forward. Maybe just float the idea of yellow flags the first time and gradually build on it as you go.

Work is a big problem to Bob. You could discuss ways around a graded return. Could treatment be specific to tasks that his work involves. Ideas of regular breaks and stretches when back. Being self employed, unless it is a large company, it is unlikely he will have any occupational health support unless he has paid for it.

CS 4.3

Is Jessie taking her medication as prescribed? Why did she believe the last treatments she had were so successful? What about them did she feel worked? Why is she stopping all activities? Has her pain actually gone away when she stops them? Often patients are not aware of these until you discuss these points.

You will often find that patients are quite reasonable when you explain all the facts to them. Not always though. At some point you may have to decide on keeping a patient happy or offering them what you know is a clinically ineffective treatment. It's a tough call. How would your manager react or support you if you refused to carry out a passive and potentially harmful (from a yellow flag psychosocial point) treatment.

Put simply, Jessie is 85. Joint pains from 'normal ageing' are very common. Patients quite like this term. They don't necessarily have 'arthritis' or 'wear and tear' but you will be surprised just how often patients are relieved to be told they are 'normal' and don't have a 'serious' illness that will put them in a wheelchair. This may help settle Jessie and get her interested in your super treatment plan. Again you will be surprised just how often patients will be delighted with explanation and often jump at the chance of taking in a self management programme.

CC 5.1

It will be sitting, bending, lifting, rising from a chair. Followed by walking, standing and lying.

If subjectively bending makes things worse (e.g. peripheralizes pain) then objectively you would expect flexion to also make leg pain worse. Think of the simple mechanics involved in most everyday movements. In most patients with LBP you should be able to reproduce the subjective answers as part of an objective assessment. In those you don't it may suggest something less mechanical.

The only way you can compare and measure outcomes is if you are measuring the same thing over and over. So many times physiotherapy departments will tweak a validated outcome measure to make it better, often invalidating an already validate questionnaire. Or for simpler outcome measures individual therapists will ask the questions in slightly different ways.

CS 5.1

There is nothing to be worried about. Yes, LBP is painful and restrictive but most people do not have one cause. This is normal, and equally frustrating. To feel less pain with a previous traumatic injury quite often is difficult for anybody to compute. You could maybe mention that his neurological testing is normal. Using the word normal is a great relaxer to patients.

There are no indicators for an X-ray. No history of trauma. Reassure Dave (and the many other real patients like him you will meet!) that guidelines discourage X-rays. They are not overly accurate in picking up much but fracture and they emit a very high dose of radiation in a sensitive area.

Dave sounds like he has already started to develop yellow flags around Beliefs and Diagnosis. Addressing them as soon as possible will help.

CC 5.2

No! I would love to be proved wrong. We can limit it and reduce the impact of it but we will never prevent it. I would love to be proved wrong but I am not holding my breath. Telling patients anything else is an untruth.

CS 6.1

1. Most likely reduced knee jerk reflex. Reduced L3 (possibly L2) in myotome amd dermatome. Reduced flexion. Maybe reduced extension too as symptoms present for 1 month so maybe starting to stiffen up in that range.
2. Fear of bending/flexion as this was mode of onset of present condition. Graded exposure, reassurance, actually addressing yellow flags with Martin.

CC 7.1

The vast majority of degenerative stenosis patients will be older, with many additional co-morbid problems. Many of these patients will have reduced spinal movement, general reduction in mobility. There may be many other medical problems that can add to a modified treatment programme. This will differ from most of your younger LBP patients who you can push on quicker and often more effectively. Also the presence of vascular problems can confuse your diagnosis.

Some things will never change; yellow flags, red flags, cauda equina etc. are all still very very relevant.

CC 8.1

All of them!!!!!!

CS 8.1

Generally you could argue yes. How does a patient still respond to pain that must be physiologically healed? But if Bob has adapted to his pain to lead a fairly normal life can there be some good from it?

John's gait pattern has adapted to allow him to work and feed his family. Almost a type of fight or flight in-built response. It is likely Bob could cause additional damage by maintaining an altered gait pattern. This needs to be addressed and dealt with.

CC 8.2

Lack of education about these medications by prescribers. I must send three patients a week back to their GP to consider supplying their patient with amitriptyline for patients who describe neurogenic pain. I have never known a GP to refuse this. Should physiotherapists have prescribing rights? We are experts in pain management.

CC 9.1

Not now it wouldn't. In the past yes. However being exposed to clinical guidelines and papers on clinically effective treatment plus clinical reasoning means I am much happier in treating LBP patients. It is quite satisfying to know that although you may not have made patients better you have offered them the best available treatment you have at hand and not offered them false hopes about treatments you know deep down won't work. The patient expects honesty too.

CC 9.3

I think physiotherapy in the past has been complicit in its own action for treating LBP in ways that will seem strange to other medical professions. However, without making me feel old, I am delighted to recognize that physiotherapy management of LBP has changed beyond recognition over the past 10 years. Days of shortwave and traction have been replaced with active treatment, back classes and returning patient to normal activities as soon as possible, often when not even pain free! Not perfect but moving in the correct direction.

CS 9.1

This is a bit like old Jessie from above. Again actually discussing previous treatments with the patient can produce satisfying results. Reviewing just how successful the exercises were that accompanied Jessie's acupuncture can produce results. Maybe she had pages of Physiotools exercises and stopped doing them all because she had a life! Picking only a few exercises and emphasizing that their main role is to facilitate 'normal' movement can be useful.

Can any Practice Educator or Senior Clinician really veto your treatment plan if it is based on a sound examination and treatment planned around clinical guidelines and a strong evidence base?

Maybe Jessie got better from having acupuncture while lying in a prone position for 30 minutes??? I look back on my junior days and think of patients I put on the super pulsed shortwave intervention taught to me over weeks at college. LBP lying prone on a plinth for 20 minutes. A lot got better. It was only when I started reflecting on these patients, reading the evidence of lack of it on LBP and shortwave and went on a McKenzie Part A course that even more patients got better on the same plinth in the same position, with the same symptoms and no flashing lights machine. Maybe Jessie just got better; LBP is quite often a self limiting condition.

The wrong approach could lead to defaulting from treatment, dissatisfied patient or developing yellow flags/chronic pain. However when push comes to shove I am an autonomous clinician who has to make a judgement on treatment I am offering based on the best available evidence. I also have a moral obligation to offer the best treatment I can to a patient. I am quite happy to use this if I need to 'refuse' to carry out what I know to be a poor treatment modality. But honesty and discussing this as an equal with a patient, rather than imposing your views on the patient, very rarely results in major confrontations.

CC 9.4

The physiotherapy management of LBP has changed. It now involves many recommendations from clinical guidelines. The evidence base on specific physiotherapy interventions is still a bit thin on the old scientific ground. As mentioned previously the physiotherapy management of LBP has changed from passive ineffective treatment, medical model of care to an active, self management, biopsychosocial strategies.

CC 9.5

In the area I practice no. But Helen's article did touch a few raw nerves, so it must happen somewhere. I remember listening to physiotherapists phoning the radio saying Helen's study was wrong, stating they gave acupuncture and massage and it did help patients. Others were offering the radio host feel pelvic realignments to prove this. Read Helen's article carefully. If you offer a thorough physiotherapy assessment coupled with evidence based advice (Back Book) then you are onto a winner. Less is sometimes more?

So long ago I can honestly not remember. I imagine when I did I was trying to promote tissue healing, reduce inflammation and take away pain.

101 different ways all with a more successful outcome to the patient.

CC 9.5

The Back Book

Index

A

Accidents, recent, 27, 91
Active straight leg raise (ASLR), 130–131
Active treatments, 162
Activity, physical, 67, 164
Acupuncture, 165, 180, 182, 221
Acute low back pain
  aims of therapy, 78–79
  European guidelines, 179–180
  management, 205
  physiotherapy-led service, 201–211
Acute pain, definition, 144–145
Adaptive pain, 149
Adherent nerve root (ANR), 125, 126, 127, 128–129
Affective pain, 153
Age of onset, 26
Agency for Health Care Policy and Research (AHCPR), US, 174
Alcohol abuse, 31
Amitriptyline, 156–157
Analgesic ladder, 154–155
Analgesics, 154–157, 179
Angina, 89
Ankle jerk reflex, 112

Assessment *see* Objective examination; Subjective examination
Attitudes, 52, 59
Audit, 46–47
Australian National Health and Medical Research Council, 174
Australian study, 200–201
Availability heuristic, 123

B

Babinski reflex, 109, 115
Back Chat, 190
Back Pain Revolution, The (Waddell), 1
Back schools, 180, 206, 208
BEAM study, 167
Bed rest, 164
Behaviours, pain, 53, 59
Beliefs, 52, 59, 65–66
Biomedical model, 163, 168
Biopsychosocial model, 163, 168
Black flags, 70, 71
Bladder problems, 87–88
Blaming trap, 96
Blood tests, 36
Blue flags, 70, 71
Body chart, 77

Bowel problems, 87–88
Breast cancer, 29–30
Bruising, 105

C

Cancer
    investigations, 34, 35, 36
    past history, 29–31, 89
    thoracic pain, 28–29
    weight loss, 32
Care pathway, traditional,
        13, 15
Case studies, 3, 213–222
Catastrophizing, 52
Cauda equina syndrome (CES),
        23, 39–49
    anatomy, 39–40
    case study, 41–43, 215
    causes, 41–43
    epidemiology, 40
    management, 210
    optimal timing of surgery,
        44–45
    pathway development, 45
    questions to ask, 87–88
    signs and symptoms, 44,
        47–49
    triage, 45–49
Central neurogenic pain, 152, 153
CES see Cauda equina syndrome
Change, readiness for, 95
Chartered Society of
        Physiotherapy, 76
Chest problems, 89
Chronic low back pain (CLBP)
    aims of therapy, 78–79
    European guidelines,
        180–181
    management, 205, 206, 209
    psychosocial risk factors see
        Psychosocial risk factors
Chronic pain, definition, 145

Classification of low back pain,
        6–7, 79
Clinical challenges, 3, 213–222
Clinical expertise, 191
Clinical guidelines, 8, 11,
        169–185
    adherence to, 171–172
    conflict with traditional
        physiotherapy, 183–184
    currently available, 173,
        174–175
    development, 170
    effectiveness, 170–171
    historical perspectives,
        173–176
    on role of physiotherapy,
        172
Clinical Standards Advisory
        Group (CSAG) manage-
        ment guidelines, 176–178
Clonus, 109, 116
Clots, blood, 89
Cochrane Database, 163,
        164–165
Cognitive dimension of pain, 148
Communication, 45–46
Community-led classes, 208
Compensation issues, 53, 59
Compliance, patient, 153
Compression test, 138
Confirmatory bias, 123–124
Confrontation/denial trap, 96
Constant pain, 27–28, 47
Control, improving, 67
Coping, 65, 148
Core Standards of Physiother-
        apy Practice (CSP), 77–78
Costs of low back pain, 10–13, 14
    direct, 11–12
    indirect, 12
    intangible, 12–13
    self-referrals, 16

Cough, pain on, 26, 47, 87
Crossed adductor reflex, 116

D

Danish Institute for Health
    and Technology
    Assessment, 174
Derangement pain, 125, 126,
    127, 128–129
Dermatomes, 112–113
DEXA scan, 90, 208
Diabetes, 90
Diagnosis
    effects of labelling, 68–69
    European Guidelines, 179,
        180
    possible errors, 124–126
    yellow flag issues, 53–54,
        59, 62–63
Diagnostic triage, 11, 22–23,
    177, 178, 214
Differential diagnosis, 103–104,
    121–141
    clinical challenges, 134,
        136, 219
    facet or zygapophyseal joint
        problems, 140
    leg pain, 124–129
    pelvic girdle pain, 128–133
    sacroiliac joint pain,
        135–140
    spinal stenosis, 133–135
Directional preference, 84
Disc prolapse, surgery, 164
Distraction test, 138
Drug abuse, intravenous
    (IVDA), 31
Drug therapy see Pharmacological
    therapy
Dual inclinometer, 106–107
Dutch College of General
    Practice, 175

E

Education, public, 200–201
Electrotherapy, 168
Emotional dimension of pain,
    148
Emotions, yellow flags, 55, 60
Employment see Work
Enhanced Back Class (EBC),
    206
Entrapment see Nerve root
    entrapment
Epilepsy, 89
European Guidelines, 173–176,
    179–181
    pelvic girdle pain, 130–133
Evidence, research, 162–163,
    167
    best, 189–190
    Cochrane reviews, 164–165
Evidence-based medicine
    (EBM), 185–191
    definition, 185–186
    in practice, 188–191, 206
Examination see Objective
    examination; Subjective
    examination
Exercise therapy, 165, 208
Expectations, patients', 69–70,
    191
Experience, previous, 64–65
Expert trap, 96
Extension, measuring, 106–107
Extension in lying exercises
    (EIL), 187

F

FABER test, 132
Facet joint problems, 140
Falls, 27, 91
Family, 55, 60
Fears, patients', 52, 68, 69
Femoral nerve stretch, 116

Finger tips to the floor test, 107
Flexion
in lying (FIL), 127, 128
measuring, 106–107
persisting severe loss, 33
in standing (DIS), 127, 128
Frequency, urinary, 44, 48–49
Functional outcome measure, 79–80

G

Gaenslen test, 131–132, 139
Gait disturbance, 88
Gender differences, 104
General practitioners (GPs), 14, 210
Greater Glasgow Back Pain Service (GGBPS), 3, 201–211
cauda equina syndrome, 45–47
effectiveness, 206–211
entry routes, 203, 205
evaluation, 203
exit routes, 205–206, 207–209
newsletter, 190
patient statistics, 204
useful statements, 67–68
yellow flag questions, 57–60

H

Health, general, 89–90
Heart disease, 89
History, 80–91
past medical, 89–90
present symptoms, 80–85
previous, 86
specific, 87–91
HIV, 31
Household productivity, 12

I

I, using, 95–97
Illusory correlation, 124
Imaging, 34–35, 205, 207
previous, 90
Inclinometer, dual, 106–107
Incontinence, 44, 48–49
Insidious onset of symptoms, 81
Interferential therapy, 181
International Association for the Study of Pain (IASP), 144–145
Intravenous drug abuse (IVDA), 31
Investigations, 34–36

J

Journal clubs, 190
Journals, 189–190

K

Kidney tumours, 29
Knee jerk reflex, 112

L

Laser treatments, 181
Laslett tests, 138–139, 140
Lateral shift, 126–127
LBP *see* Low back pain
Leeds Assessment of Neuropathic Symptoms and Signs (S-LANSS), 157
Leg pain, differential diagnosis, 124–129
Legal issues, 53, 59
Listening, reflective, 97–99
Lordosis, 105
Low back pain (LBP)
definition, 6
terminology, 3
Lower motor neuron lesions, 108, 109

Lumbago, 54
Lung cancer, 29

M

Magnetic resonance imaging (MRI), 35, 205, 207
Maladaptive pain, 149
Manipulation therapy, 165, 167
McKenzie Diagnosis and Therapy (MDT), 127, 187
Mechanical pain, 27
Media, mass, 183–184, 200–201, 222
Medical history, past, 89–90
Medication see Pharmacological therapy
Metastases, 29–30
Motor pain, 152–153
Movement
    exaggerated response, 105
    mechanics, 103
    range of, 105–107
Multi-segmental involvement, 109
Muscle relaxants, 155
Muscle spasm, 105
Myotomes, 113, 114, 115

N

National Health and Medical Research Council, Australia, 174
Nerve root entrapment, 54, 68
    differential diagnosis, 125, 126, 127, 128
    management, 205
Netherlands College of General Practice, 175
Neurological abnormalities, multiple, 32, 48
Neurological examination, 107–116

Neuropathic/neurogenic pain, 152, 153, 155–156
Neurosurgeon, 45–46
New Zealand National Advisory Committee on Health and Disability, 174
Night pain, 28, 91
Nociceptive pain, 151, 154–155
Non-mechanical pain, 27–28, 47
Non-steroidal anti-inflammatory drugs (NSAIDs), 155, 179, 180
Numerical rating scale (NRS), 78–79

O

Objective examination, 101–118
    case study, 116–117, 219
    clinical challenge, 105
    leg pain, 126–127
    reliability, 117
Observation, 104
Occupational flags, 71
Opioids, 155–156, 180
Orthopaedic surgeon, 13, 205, 207
Osteoporosis, 34, 90, 208, 210
Outcome measures, 77–80
Overconfidence, 123

P

Paediatric cases, 210
Pain, 143–158
    adaptive and maladaptive, 149
    case study, 149–150, 219
    clinical challenges, 145, 150, 219, 220
    definition, 144–145
    dimensions, 147–148
    epidemiology, 145–146
    mechanisms, 151–153
    natural history, 146–147

Pain Association Scotland (PAS), 209
Pain clinics, 209
Pain rating scales, 78–79
Paracetamol, 179
Passive interventions, 162
Past medical history (PMH), 89–90
Pathway of care, traditional, 13, 15
Patient satisfaction, 206
Pelvic girdle pain (PGP), 128–133
Peripheral neurogenic pain, 152
Pharmacological therapy, 153–157
    clinical challenge, 156, 218
    clinical guidelines, 179, 180
    costs, 11, 12
    history, 88
    non-compliance, 153
Physical activity, 67, 164
Physical therapies, 180
Physiotherapy
    changing role, 13–16, 39
    led back pain service, 201–211
Plantar (Babinski) reflex, 109, 115
Posterior pelvic pain provocation test, 132–133
Posture
    sitting, 104
    standing, 126–127
Pregnancy, pelvic girdle pain, 130
Premature focus trap, 97
Prevention, 181
Prodigy Guidelines, 11, 173–176, 178–179, 181
Progressive pain, 27
Prostate cancer, 29
Psychology, 206

Psychosocial risk factors, 52–56, 59–60, 164
    see also Yellow flags

Q
Quality Improvement Scotland, 172
Quebec Task Force on Spinal Disorders, 79
Question/answer trap, 96
Questions, 91–95
    closed, 92
    contextualizing, 93–95
    leading, 92–93
    open, 92

R
Randomized controlled trials (RCTs), 162–163
Range of movement, 105–107
RCGP see Royal College of General Practitioners
Recurrence of low back pain, 7–9
Red flags, 21–36, 67
    cauda equina syndrome, 47–49
    clinical challenges, 23, 31, 33, 34, 214–215
    common, 25–33
    investigations, 34–36
    prevalence, 33–34
    questions to ask, 87–91
    requiring emergency referral, 23
    significance of individual, 23–25
Referrals, 13, 15, 205, 207
Referred leg pain, differential diagnosis, 124–129
Reflective listening, 97–99
Reflexes, 109, 111–112
Representativeness heuristic, 122–123

Return to work (RTW), 68, 216, 217
Rheumatoid arthritis, 89
Road traffic accidents, recent, 27
Royal College of General Practitioners (RCGP) guidelines, 11, 173–176, 178

S

Sacral thrust, 139
Sacroiliac joint (SIJ) pain, 135–140
Saddle anaesthesia, 44, 48–49
Schrober's index, 106
Sciatica, 54, 68
Self care, 205, 208
Self-referral, 16–17, 39
Sensory dimension of pain, 148
Serious spinal pathology (SSP), 22, 33–34, 67
    management, 210
    significance of red flags, 23–25
    see also Red flags
Services, specialist, 199–211
Severe LBP problems, 102
Sitting posture, 104
Sleep disturbance, 85
Sneezing, pain on, 26, 47, 87
Social security benefits, 10–11
Spasm, muscle, 105
Spinal cord compression (SCC), malignant, 28–29, 29, 30
Spinal manipulation, 165, 167
Spinal pathology, serious see Serious spinal pathology
Spinal stenosis, 133–135, 219
Standing posture, 126–127
Steroid use, long-term, 31
Stork test, 132
Straight leg raise (SLR), 110–111
    active (ASLR), 130–131

Stroke, 89
Subjective examination, 75–100
    avoiding traps, 95–97
    case study, 82, 218
    clinical challenges, 80, 82, 85, 93, 94, 217–218
    history taking, 80–91
    leg pain, 125–126
    outcome measures, 77–80
    questions, 91–95
    reflective listening, 97–99
    starting point, 76–77
Substance abuse, 31
Surgery, 164, 207
    past history, 90–91
Sympathetic pain, 152–153
Symphysis pain
    palpation test, 133
    provocation test, 132
Symptoms
    change over time, 84
    duration, 80
    factors aggravating/easing, 84
    intermittent vs constant, 83
    means of onset, 81
    at onset of current episode, 82–83
    present, 77, 80–85
    previous, 86
Systematic reviews, 162–163, 164–165
Systemic illness, 31–32

T

Take home messages, 4
Thigh thrust, 132–133, 138
Thoracic pain, 28–29
Traction, lumbar, 181
Transcutaneous electrical nerve stimulation (TENS), 165, 180, 181
Traps, during assessment, 95–97

Trauma
    onset of LBP, 81
    previous history, 27, 47, 91
    signs, 105
Treatment, 161–192
    active, 162
    case study, 182, 220–221
    clinical challenges, 166, 171,
        172, 183, 184, 220–222
    goals, 9, 95
    physiotherapy consensus,
        167–168
    previous, 86
    provided in practice, 168–169
    readiness for, 95
    sources of guidance, 169–185
    traditional physiotherapy,
        162–167, 183–184
    yellow flag issues, 53–54,
        59, 70
Trendelenburg's test, modified,
    132
Triage
    cauda equina syndrome,
        45–49
    diagnostic, 11, 22–23,
        177, 214
Tricyclic antidepressants, 155,
    156–157

U

Ultrasound (U/S) therapy, 181,
    187
Unemployment benefits, 10
United States Agency for Health
        Care Policy and Research
        (AHCPR), 174
Upper limb involvement, 109
Upper motor neuron disorders,
    108, 109
Urinalysis, 36
Urinary retention, 44, 48–49
Urological symptoms, 48–49

V

Values, patients', 191
Vascular symptoms, 134
Vertebroplasty, 210
Visual analogue scale (VAS), 78–79

W

Weakness, 109
Weight loss, 32
Work
    blue and black flags, 70, 71
    costs of LBP, 10–11, 12
    onset of LBP at, 81
    return to, 68, 216, 217
    yellow flags, 55–56, 60, 71
Working Backs Scotland, 200
World Health Organization
        (WHO), analgesic ladder,
        154–155

X

X-rays, 34–35, 205, 207

Y

Yellow flags, 51–72
    ABCDEFW, 52–56, 59–60
    case studies, 56–57, 61–62,
        63–64, 215–217
    checklist of questions, 57–60
    clinical challenges, 57, 60,
        66, 214–215
    clinical guidelines, 173
    definition, 52
    evidence-based practice, 190
    identification, 52–61, 103
    management, 62–65, 206
    other associated flags, 70–71
    possible interventions, 65–70
    suggested words/phrases, 70

Z

Zygapophyseal joint problems,
    140